Johnson's First Aid Manual

THE CLASSIC 1929 EDITION

EDITED BY FREDERICK B. KILMER

CLYDESDALE

First published in 1914 by Johnson & Johnson

First Clydesdale Press Edition 2018

All rights to any and all materials in copyright owned by the publisher are strictly reserved by the publisher.

Clydesdale books may be purchased in bulk at special discounts for sales promotion, corporate gifts, fund-raising, or educational purposes. Special editions can also be created to specifications. For details, contact the Special Sales Department, Skyhorse Publishing, 307 West 36th Street, 11th Floor, New York, NY 10018 or info@skyhorsepublishing.com.

Clydesdale Press™ is a pending trademark of Skyhorse Publishing, Inc.®, a Delaware corporation.

Visit our website at www.skyhorsepublishing.com.

10 9 8 7 6 5 4 3 2 1

Library of Congress Cataloging-in-Publication Data is available on file.

Print ISBN: 978-1-945186-42-4
eISBN: 978-1-945186-43-1

Printed in the United States of America

COLLABORATORS

In the Revision of this Manual the Editor has had the Assistance and Valued Suggestions of a Large Number of Workers in the Field of First Aid Among Whom are the Following:

MR. JOHN L. BOARDMAN
Chairman, Bureau of Safety, Anaconda Copper Mining Company, Butte, Montana

DR. WALTER M. BRICKNER
Lieut.-Colonel, Medical Reserve Corps, U.S.A.; Surgeon, New York City

CAPTAIN CLARENCE E. BURT, M. D.
Medical Corps, United States Army (retired), New Bedford, Mass.

DR. D. P. BUSH
Medical and Sanitary Officer, Government Printing Office, Washington, D. C.

MR. H. CALL
General Organizer, First Aid, Canadian National Railways, Toronto, Ontario, Canada

DR. W. IRVING CLARK
Service Director, Norton Company, Worcester, Mass.

DR. ALBERT N. CROUCH
Medical Director, American Locomotive Company, Schenectady, N. Y.

DR. THOMAS R. CROWDER
Director, Department Sanitation and Surgery, Pullman Company, Chicago, Ill.

DR. H. L. DAIELL
Research Division, Johnson & Johnson, New Brunswick, N. J.

MARION L. DANNENBERG
Formerly Director of Health Education of the Henry Phipps Institute, University of Pennsylvania, Philadelphia, Pa.

COMMODORE WILLIAM J. DAVIDS
U. S. Life Saving Corps, Long Beach, Calif.

DR. GEORGE G. DAVIS
Chief Surgeon, Illinois Steel Company, Chicago, Ill.

DR. WILLARD J. DENNO
Medical Director, Standard Oil Company, New York City

MR. S. C. DICKINSON
Safety Engineer, Pacific Gas & Electric Company, San Francisco, Calif.

MR. JAMES B. DOUGLAS
Manager Insurance Department, The United Gas Improvement Company, Philadelphia, Pa.

DR. G. G. DOWDALL
Chief Surgeon, Illinois Central Railroad Company, Chicago, Ill.

DR. W. A. EVANS
Health Department, Chicago Tribune, Chicago, Ill.

FIDELITY & CASUALTY COMPANY
New York City

MR. C. D. FISHER
First Aid Instructor, Pennsylvania Railroad Company Y. M. C. A., Camden, N. J.

DR. F. M. FURLONG
Medical Director, American Radiator Company, Buffalo, N. Y.

MR. S. A. GIDLOW
Instructor, St. John's Ambulance Association, Montreal, Canada

DR. H. LYNN HALBERT
United States Gypsum Company, ot. George, Staten Island, New York City

MR. THOMAS E. HICKS
First Aid Division, Johnson & Johnson, New Brunswick, N. J.

DR. H. F. HOFFMEIER
Chief Surgeon, Central Railroad of New Jersey, Mauch Chunk, Pa.

P. D. I. HONEYMAN
Metallurgist, International Smelting Company, Inspiration, Arizona

DR. W. RANDOLPH HURST, F.A.C.S.
District Surgeon, Louisville & Nashville Railroad, Evansville, Indiana

DR. E. H. INGRAM
Plant Physician, The William Cramp & Sons Ship & Engine Building Company, Philadelphia, Pa.

{ 3 }

Collaborators (*continued*)

DR. ELMER CHASE JACKSON
Works Physician, Medical Advisory Commission, Incandescent Lamp Department, General Electric Company, Harrison, N. J.

COL. RICHARD P. KELLY
Supt., Palo Alto Military Academy, Palo Alto, Calif.

DR. R. T. LEGGE
University Physician, Professor of Hygiene, University of California, Berkeley, Calif.

DR. WILL F. LYON
Chicago, Ill.

DR. DAVID TRUMBULL MARSHALL
Hollis, Long Island, New York

DR. CARY P. McCORD
Medical Director, Industrial Health Conservancy Laboratories, Cincinnati, Ohio

DR. GEORGE B. MORELAND, F.A.C.S.,
Pittsburgh, Pa.

DR. H. S. MURAT
American Rolling Mill Company Hospital, Middletown, Ohio

CAPTAIN PIKE
General Secretary, Queensland Ambulance Transport Brigade, Ann Street, Brisbane, Australia

DR. E. H. REBHORN
Scranton, Pa.

DR. F. L. RECTOR
Editor, *Nation's Health*, Chicago, Ill.

DR. R. D. RICHMAN
Medical Advisor, Aetna Life Insurance Company, Aetna Casualty & Surety Company, Automobile Insurance Company of Hartford, Conn., Hartford, Conn.

DR. R. R. SAYERS
Chief Surgeon, U. S. Bureau of Mines, Surgeon U. S. Public Health Service, Dept. of Commerce, Bureau of Mines, Washington, D. C.

DR. F. E. SCHUBMEHL
Works Physician, General Electric Company, West Lynn, Mass.

MR. EMIL J. SENNE
Vacuum Oil Company, New York City

DR. JAMES WARREN SEVER
Surgeon at Children's Hospital, Boston, Mass.

MR. A. G. SHAKESPEARE
First Aid Department, Canadian Pacific Railway, Montreal, Canada

DR. H. S. SHARPE, C.M., F.A.C.S.
Lecturer in First Aid, Brandon, Manitoba, Canada

DR. LOYAL A. SHOUDY
Chief Surgeon, Bethlehem Steel Company, Inc., Bethlehem, Pa.

MR. C. C. THOMAS
Superintendent, Van Buren Schools, Marion, Indiana

DR. L. R. THOMPSON
Surgeon in Charge, United States Public Health Service, Washington, D. C.

UNITED GAS IMPROVEMENT CO.
Philadelphia, Pa.

UNITED STATES INDUSTRIAL ALCOHOL COMPANY
New York, N. Y.

DR. A. J. VAN BRUNT
Director Safety Education, Public Service Corporation of New Jersey, Newark, N. J.

DR. RALPH F. WARD, F.A.C.S.
Attending Surgeon, Chief of Service, Metropolitan Hospital, Department of Public Welfare, City of New York; Major Medical Officers Reserve Corps, U. S. A., New York City

DR. F. C. WARNSHUIS
Grand Rapids, Mich.

DR. EARL H. WELCOME
Lieutenant Colonel, Medical Reserves United States Army, Industrial Surgeon, Downey, California

MR. J. W. WEST, JR.
Secretary Accident Prevention Committee, American Gas Association, New York City

MISS SARAH O. WHITLOCK
Principal, Lord Sterling School, New Brunswick, N. J.

DR. IRA S. WILE
First Aid Lecturer and Writer, New York City

DR. R. C. WILLIAMS
Assistant Surgeon General, Bureau Public Health Service, Washington, D. C.

PROF. ADOLPH ZIEFLE
Dean, Oregon State Agricultural College, Corvallis, Oregon

PREFACE TO THE TENTH REVISION

IN PREPARING this new and thoroughly revised edition of the Manual, the editor has been fortunate in receiving the suggestions of specialists, representative surgeons, physicians, first aid teachers and workers of long experience in railway, mining, police and industrial service in this country and abroad, some of whose names are elsewhere noted. The Manual now reflects the opinion of the whole field of first aid in a way that makes for uniformity in methods and materials and common rules of practice for all ordinary emergencies. It standardizes first aid.

All of the characteristic features of previous editions which have stood the test of practical experience and professional criticism and have won popular approval are retained. New information brought to light by the rapid development of the practice of the art of first aid has been added. The entire text has been rewritten, reedited and reset. New illustrations have been made from living models, under the direction of trained workers.

The suggestions given in the Manual are not intended to be elaborate. Extensiveness has been sacrificed to simplicity. Much that is usually found in works of this character has been omitted, and only that believed to be the most simple, essential and helpful has been selected. No attempt has been made to teach anatomy or physiology, or to give instruction in the principles and practice of surgery.

Technical terms have been avoided. Everything is placed before the reader in the simplest and plainest form.

Thus the work becomes more than ever a standard First Aid Manual for everyday use and from it any one who can read English or understand a picture may gain information which will serve in emergency.

WHAT IS FIRST AID?

FIRST AID to the injured has been aptly described as a bridge between the accident and medical or surgical assistance, and over this bridge the injured person is to be carried from the place of injury to a place of treatment.

Such action is first aid whoever may render it. A person trained in first aid, a physician or a nurse, may render more skillful aid than one who is untrained, but in every instance the action is first aid.

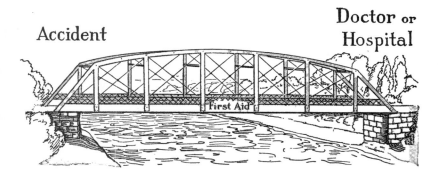

Once the bridge is crossed, and the injured person in the hands of the medical attendant (or hospital), first aid is at an end.

First aid teachers, workers and trainers are apt to go beyond the scope and limit of true first aid as here outlined. The treatment and care of injuries, the administration of medicines, the diagnosis and treatment of disease are no part of first aid work.

It is undoubtedly a mistake for first aid teachers to attempt to train workers in anatomy or physiology, except when limited to the most elementary phases; certainly it is far outside the principles of first aid to attempt the treatment of disease, the after-care of wounds, the setting of fractures and like measures.

First aid work now involves the prevention of the spread of contagion, relief in sudden sickness and other emergencies.

HOW TO USE THE MANUAL

THIS Manual is designed as a working Manual in first aid, and is arranged in such a manner that any particular subject can be quickly referred to in an emergency. The possessor of the Manual, however, should not wait for an accident to occur before testing the value of these instructions, or his own ability to carry them out.

Those who are likely to be called upon to take care of the injured should familiarize themselves with this book, as well as with the materials which are to be applied. To this end it is suggested that the book be read through, noting the general principles that govern first aid. This should be followed by a more careful study of the suggestions and details, and an attempt made to impress the more important points upon the memory.

The student should particularly study the methods which apply to his own calling in life.

Designedly, no instructions are given in this Manual in respect to anatomy or physiology. A knowledge of these subjects is not considered as essential, either to the intelligent use of the Manual or to the application of first aid. The reader who may have occasion to practice first aid as a calling is, however, advised to secure, on the recommendation of a physician, some simple text-book upon these subjects. The general direction of the main arteries, and the location of the points where the circulation may be arrested by pressure may be learned by a study of the illustrations in this Manual. The reader is urged to determine upon himself, or better still, upon a companion, the location of main points where pressure is to be applied in cases of bleeding. He should also be able to locate the principal parts of the skeleton which are liable to become fractured.

Practice makes perfect. Therefore, the reader will be greatly benefited if he will procure a supply of the dressings and some of the appliances suggested in the Manual, and actually use them. He can practice upon himself or secure the aid of friends to act as patients. Bandages or other articles used for practice purposes should never be applied to a wound; they should be used for practice only. Familiarity with the contents and use of articles contained in First Aid outfits is of prime importance.

In factories, mines, shops, and places of like character, the Manual and all first aid material should be placed in charge of the superintendent, foreman, or some person who is likely to be constantly on duty. The Manual should be kept in a conspicuous place, in order that it may be the first thing found in emergency.

All material to be used for first aid purposes should be kept in a closed box, or closet. Unnecessary handling of first aid material should be avoided. All dressings to be applied to wounds should be such as are known to be surgically clean and aseptic, and should be kept in the original sealed package.

The instructions and illustrations given in this book are such as will apply to dressings and material which may be procured at any drug store. Directions for the preparation of home-made appliances are included, as well as suggestions for the use of material that is likely to be found at any place where an accident may occur.

The layman into whose hands this Manual may fall should ever bear in mind the oft-repeated injunction: "Send for a physician." However great or small may be the emergency, nothing can take the place of a physician. "A little knowledge is a dangerous thing." "Beware of an axe in the hands of a child." All of the first aid manuals ever printed, if taken together, would not transform a layman into a surgeon. Hence it is of prime importance that the layman shall acquire the art of knowing when to cease all attempts at first aid and place the patient in the hands of a physician.

Principles of First Aid

The first aid student should be:

Observant, noting the cause and signs of injury.

Tactful, that he may avoid thoughtless questions and learn the symptoms and history of the case.

Resourceful, using to the best advantage whatever is at hand to prevent further damage.

Explicit, giving clear instructions to the patient and advice to the assistants.

Discriminating, that he may decide which of the several injuries should be first given attention.

THE FIRST THINGS TO DO

B E CALM. Send for a physician at once. When possible, write a brief message describing the accident and injury, so the physician may know what instruments and remedies to bring.

Assume command of the situation. There can be only one chief.

Give first aid treatment as soon as possible. Keep bystanders away. Give the victim room to breathe. If possible and safe, remove the patient to a quiet, airy place, where the temperature is moderate; never to a hot room. Handle the patient firmly but gently.

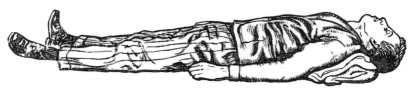

Fig. 1—Injured patient with head slightly lower than body.

Place the injured person in a comfortable position, preferably on his back. Loosen the collar, waist-band and belt. Straighten the limbs out in their natural position, preferably with the toes up. Injuries to the head may require that it be raised higher than the level of the body. If breathing is difficult, a semi-sitting position is best. If the patient be faint, let his head be lower than his feet. In cases of fracture "splint where they lie" before moving.

Watch the patient carefully, if he be unconscious.

If vomiting occurs, turn the patient's head on one side and

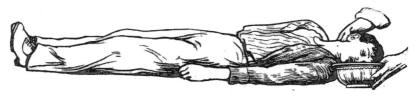

Fig. 2—Turning the patient's head to relieve vomiting.

raise the shoulder so as to keep the mouth clear of vomited food.

If a wound be discovered in a part covered by the clothing, cut the clothing in the seam, so as to permit bandaging the wound. In case of burns the adhering clothing should be cut away with scissors, do not attempt to remove by pulling forcibly.

Dress all wounds as quickly as possible. (See instructions elsewhere in this Manual.) If severe bleeding should occur, stop it before the wound is dressed.

After dressing a wound, do only what is absolutely necessary to transport the patient to a place of safety.

SHOCK OR COLLAPSE

Shock is common after serious accidents.

Do not allow a person to see his own injury, especially bleeding. It may provoke shock.

The signs of shock are a cool, clammy skin, vomiting and retching, weak, rapid pulse, sighing or irregular breathing, half-opened eyelids, dilated pupils, dullness of mind, and sometimes insensibility or coma with skin of gray or greenish hue. Send for a physician at once.

Place the patient in a warm bed or wrap him in blankets or coats. Keep his head low. Bind up wounds and splint broken bones.

Apply heat, especially to the region of the heart, the pit of the stomach and to the extremities. Use bottles of hot water, rubber water-bags, hot bricks, or blankets and flannels wrung out of hot water, in fact anything hot that may be convenient. Be careful that applications are not too hot, test them on your cheek. Wrap hot articles in blankets so as not to burn the skin. Apply heat along the inner sides of the arms and legs. Do not apply heat to the head. Do not give hot drinks in brain injuries, nor in severe bleeding.

Hot water, tea, coffee, broth or hot milk are the best stimulants. Do not give whisky, brandy, or other spirituous liquors. If patient is able to swallow, one-half teaspoonful of aromatic spirit of ammonia in half a cup of water every fifteen minutes for not more than four doses may be given if necessary. Do not give stimulants while patient remains unconscious.

Relieve vomiting by placing bits of cracked ice in the patient's mouth. In summer, let the injured person sip cold water if he is conscious.

BLEEDING

Summon a physician at once. Have the patient lie down, usually on his back. If the wound is in a limb, elevate it. Cut away clothing (following seams) to expose and examine the wound. Stop the bleeding.

First aid ends when the bleeding is stopped and the wound covered with a bandage. Do not give stimulants until bleeding has stopped.

Arterial Bleeding (from the arteries).—Arterial bleeding is very dangerous and may destroy life in a few minutes. Arterial blood is bright red—scarlet—spurting. When in doubt, treat all bleeding as arterial.

To control—Cover your thumb with several thicknesses of clean gauze or soft cloths and press directly on the wound, to stop bleeding temporarily. If the wound is large, cover with a pad made with thick layers of gauze or other material. Then apply pressure at a short distance above the spurting point, (between the wound and the heart). If the bleeding does not stop, apply a tourniquet, made with the triangular bandage, a pair of suspenders, a piece of rubber tubing, the inner tube of an automobile, or a piece of rope. *A tourniquet left on too long may induce gangrene. Any sort of tourniquet should be loosened at least every twenty minutes by the clock to allow circulation to return; oftener, if part becomes cold or dark. If bleeding starts, tighten again.*

If a limb is badly crushed, put the pressure on the limb above the crushed tissues.

Fit the pressure bandage firmly before leaving it. After the bleeding has been stopped, remove the bandage slowly and apply another bandage that will not obstruct the circulation of the part.

Venous Bleeding (from the veins).—Venous blood flows toward the heart, is dark red or purplish, wells up freely without spurting.

To control—Lay a pad of dry gauze over the wound and bind up with a moderately firm bandage.

In severe cases have the patient lie down. Elevate the wounded part, loosen tight clothing, collars, waistbands and other constricting garments. Apply a pressure pad below the bleeding point, between the wound and the end of the extremity. Pad the wound with gauze, and bandage.

Cuts of the throat, involving the jugular vein, are the most dangerous. (See Bleeding from Special Parts, pages 13-18.)

Ruptures of the varicose veins of the legs are common. In these, elevate the limb, remove garters, and bandage the leg firmly below the wound, and then place a small compress directly upon the opening.

Oozing from wounds, capillary bleeding, occurs in nearly every variety of small wounds. Exposure to the air for a few moments will often allow clotting and check this form of bleeding. Hot water applied by means of squeezing out a mass of hot cloths is sometimes successful. (Warm water encourages bleeding.) Extremely cold water or a piece of ice also checks bleeding. Usually it is sufficient to apply a pad of gauze upon the bleeding part and to bind it tightly in place. If the bleeding be from the socket of a tooth, it may be controlled by packing the cavity with bits of cotton or gauze.

Bleeding: General Treatment—In every form of bleeding, keep the patient warm by artificial heat and clothing, hot water bags, etc.

When the bleeding has ceased, give hot drinks, tea, coffee, milk, etc., and cautiously loosen the bandages if they are tight.

Keep watch for recurrence of the bleeding. When it occurs, tighten the bandages or apply pressure as before.

Severe bleeding may cause fainting; this may temporarily check the bleeding. Treat as any other fainting spell. Lay the patient upon the floor or couch, lower the head, keep the limbs elevated, apply warmth to the body. Be ready to check

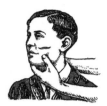

Fig. 3—To arrest bleeding of the cheek.

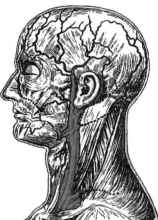

Fig. 5—Course of the main arteries of the face, neck and scalp.

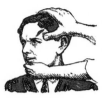

Fig. 6—To arrest bleeding of the temple.

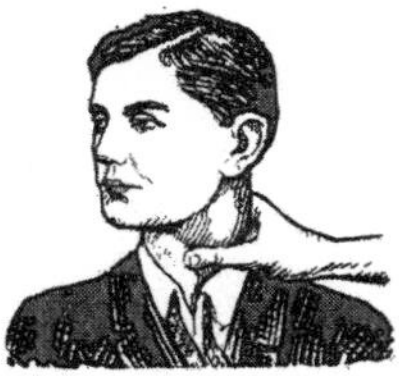

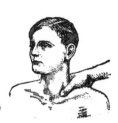

Fig. 4—To arrest bleeding of the neck.

Fig. 7—To arrest bleeding of the upper part of the arm or armpit.

the bleeding again if it should recur when consciousness is restored.

BLEEDING FROM SPECIAL PARTS

Scalp—Press down directly upon the scalp near the edge of the wound, on the side from which the bleeding proceeds (Fig. 8). Make a permanent compress by folding gauze cloth into a hard pad and bind it firmly. (See Bandaging.)

Temple—Press with the thumb upon the bone just in front of the ear, to compress the artery. (Fig. 6.)

Make a permanent compress by means of a piece of plain gauze folded in the form of a pad, and hold it in place with a roller or triangular bandage. (See Bandaging.)

Face—Press firmly against the jaw bone with the thumb. (Fig. 3.) Control bleeding of the cheek and lips by passing the thumb into the patient's mouth and grasping the cheek, just below the wound, between the thumb and the fingers, thus compressing the artery leading to the wound. (Fig. 9.) Bind a folded piece of gauze as a permanent pad compress. (See Bandaging.)

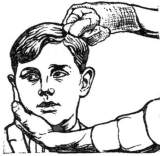

Fig. 8—To arrest bleeding of the scalp. Pressure applied directly to the bleeding point with the thumb, the thumb covered with clean cloth or gauze.

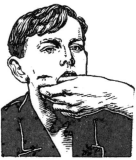

Fig. 9—To arrest bleeding from the cheek. Pressure applied by placing the thumb inside the mouth and the finger outside.

Neck—Stab wounds, cut throat or other wounds of this region require prompt attention. Without an instant's delay, grasp the patient's neck. (Fig. 4.) Put the thumb into the wound and press the wounded vessels straight back against the spine and not against the wind pipe. Continue the thumb pressure until assistance arrives.

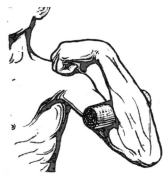

Fig. 10—Flexion of the arm at the elbow to arrest bleeding. A piece of wood or hard substance thrust inside the elbow. The arm may be fastened in this position.

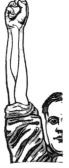

Fig. 11—Elevation of the arm with the hand grasping a hard substance.

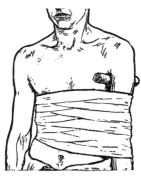

Fig. 12—Compression to arrest bleeding of axillary artery (armpit). A piece of wood (or book) thrust into the space and the arm bandaged to the side.

Arm—If the arm is not entirely severed, roll a towel about a bottle or other hard, round substance, or tie a hard knot in a towel, and crowd it into the armpit. A roll of news-paper, or stick of wood, or other hard substance covered with sterile gauze, may be utilized. (Fig. 12.) Then bring the arm to the side and fasten firmly with the bandage. If the bleeding is in the armpit, make pressure with a pad of sterile gauze directly upon the bleeding point. If the arm is severed, press upon the artery on the first rib just back of the collar bone, with the thumb or fingers (Fig. 7) or with a padded key.

Arterial bleeding in the arm may be checked as described above, or pressure may be applied, as shown in Fig. 15. A Spanish windlass tourniquet, or a bandage applied to the arm (Fig. 17) with a wad or pad covering the wound, may be used in addition, or to relieve the pressure.

Forearm and Wrist—Raise the forearm above the head. (Fig. 11.) In addition to the pressure on the wound, or above it, place a hard object, such as a small bottle or stick, in the front of the elbow, then bend the forearm at the elbow and bandage firmly to the upper-arm. (Fig. 10.)

Palm of the Hand—Raise the arm above the head. Have the patient grasp some small, hard object like a billiard ball or smooth stone, covered with sterile gauze. The pressure may be made permanent by binding the hand firmly while in this position. (Fig. 11.)

Fingers—Raise the arm above the head. Apply pressure to the hand or wrist by binding with a pad and bandage. No violent pressure is needed.

Chest and Abdomen—Apply pressure upon the wound itself. If available take a yard of surgical gauze, crumple it up and press it into the wound until the physician arrives, or keep it in place by applying a firm bandage around the body.

Bleeding from the Lungs—(Blood bright red, sometimes light coffee color.) Lay the patient down with head and shoulders raised.

Summon a physician at once. Keep patient absolutely quiet and cool, applying cold, wet cloths to the chest.
Give finely chopped ice.

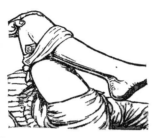

Fig. 13—Flexion of the knee to arrest bleeding in the leg or foot. A piece of wood to be inserted under the knee, the leg bent back upon itself and fastened with a bandage.

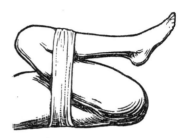

Fig. 14—Flexion of the leg to arrest bleeding in the thigh. A stick or knotted cloth placed in the groin and the leg bent back upon the abdomen and fastened with a bandage.

Bleeding from the Stomach—(Blood, dark coffee color.) Give ice water or broken ice with a teaspoonful of vinegar, repeating the dose at intervals. Summon a physician at once.

Internal Bleeding—Lay the patient upon a bed or couch without a pillow, with the head slightly lower than the body. Apply ice-cold cloths to the abdomen. A surgeon should always be summoned.

Bleeding from the Tongue—If severe, apply pressure as for bleeding of the arteries of the neck. Let the patient suck ice or sip very hot water.

Bleeding from the Nose—Apply cold cloths or cracked ice over nose and at the back of the neck.

Have patient sit erect with head dropped slightly forward.

Pinch nostrils together and hold for a few minutes.

A simple method is placing under the upper lip a small wad of cotton or gauze and applying pressure up against the nose.

If bleeding persists, take a narrow strip of gauze and crowd a small portion at a time into the nostril, pushing it well up into nose with a pencil or penholder until a tight plug is produced.

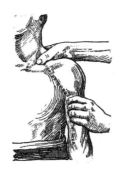

Fig. 15—To arrest bleeding of the upper arm.

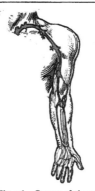

Fig. 16—Course of the main arteries in the arm and shoulder.

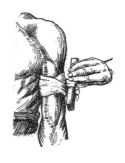

Fig. 17—Spanish windlass applied to the arm.

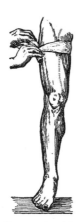

Fig. 18—Spanish windlass to arrest bleeding of the artery of the thigh.

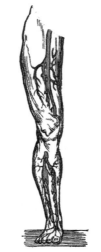

Fig. 19—Course of the main arteries of the leg.

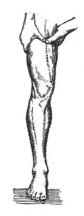

Fig. 20—Hand-pressure to arrest bleeding in the leg or thigh.

Keep plug in nose several hours, and when bleeding has stopped remove carefully so as not to renew the bleeding.

If bleeding is excessive or continuous, summon a physician.

Thigh—Thigh wounds require prompt attention. Exert pressure upon the inner surface of the thigh just below the groin, or where the artery of the thigh (femoral artery) comes out of

[17]

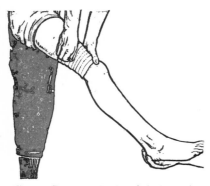

Fig. 21—To arrest bleeding of the leg or foot. The limb elevated and pressure applied by means of a bandage.

the body, about two-thirds of the way from the knee to the hipjoint. (Fig. 20.) This can be effected with the thumbs, a rounded stick, a key handle, or a Spanish windlass. (Fig. 18.) To control the artery, place a knotted cloth or a large round stone in the groin, doubling the leg back on the thigh (this is important); press the thigh up against the abdomen; finally, hold it there with a bandage. (Fig. 14.)

A piece of elastic tubing (inner tube of an automobile tire) or a pair of suspenders passed around the limb several times, stretched at each turning and made tight, is often effective. Draw only tight enough to control bleeding. Loosen every twenty minutes and retighten if bleeding is not checked.

Leg Below the Knee—Apply firm pressure in the hollow just behind the knee above the calf of the leg. Place a stick under the knee and double the leg back until it presses hard against it. (Fig. 13.) Pressure may also be applied as shown in Fig. 21.

Spanish Windlass—This is a rough but effective method of controlling bleeding in the arms or legs, and should be used only where other methods fail or cannot be carried out. Its construction and application are shown in Figs. 17 and 18. Use only as a temporary expedient in an emergency and for no longer time than is necessary to check the bleeding. It should be loosened every fifteen minutes and re-tightened. As soon as it is safe to do so remove and substitute a flat pad.

Bleeding from the Foot—Apply pressure to the bleeding point, or to the arteries at the ankle joint. If this fails, use flexion of the knee. (Fig. 13.)

WOUNDS

Summon a physician. Place the patient in a comfortable position while the wound is being examined and dressed. Stop the bleeding. (See Bleeding, pages 11-18). Cleanse your hands with soap and water and cover the finger with surgical gauze or lint before touching the wound.

In accidents, every wound is likely to become contaminated with dirt and foreign substances, which hinder the healing of the wound. Do not attempt to cleanse the wound if the services of a physician can be obtained. It is safer, as a rule, to bind up the wound temporarily, dirt and all, than to touch it with unclean hands. Cover the wound as quickly as possible with the cleanest material available. Small wounds such as scratches, pin pricks, etc., should be cared for the same as the larger ones.

Iodine on Wounds—Solutions of iodine are extensively used as an application to wounds to prevent infection. They should be applied with caution. The tincture of iodine as purchased in drug stores, should not be used full strength. It should be reduced to at least half strength with alcohol.

Solutions of iodine increase in strength upon standing, owing to the evaporation of the solvent. Old solutions are liable to irritate and even produce blisters, they should be reduced in strength with alcohol.

Solutions of iodine of proper strength for application to wounds are now supplied in first aid kits. These may be obtained in tubes or in ampoules with a swab attached for applying the solution.

Iodine should be applied as soon as possible after the injury, and with a swab made of cotton or gauze, wiping off any excess, and allowing it to dry. It should not be poured into a wound.

Iodine should not be applied to the eye, the nose, the mouth or the throat. Iodine should be used with caution on the aged and the very young. Solutions of iodine should not be poured over bandages.

Iodine must always be used with due caution.

Mercurochrome—Solutions of mercurochrome have come into use as a substitute for iodine for application to wounds. These solutions are usually supplied two per cent strength. Solutions of mercurochrome form a part of many first aid equipments, they are also obtainable in tubes or ampoules with swabs attached for applying the solutions.

Mercurochrome solutions stain the skin an orange red. They are non-irritating and may be used with safety.

Mercurochrome, like iodine, is to be painted over and around the wound, not poured on.

In cases where there is grease or other foreign substances, the area around the wound, but not the wound itself, may be cleaned with gasoline or benzine.

Pick dirt, bits of grass or clothing, splinters of wood, fish-hooks, pins or thorns out of the wound with tweezer or pincers that have been first boiled in water.

Before replacing any of the torn portions of the wound, wash your hands thoroughly, cover your hand with surgical gauze or lint, as with a glove. Do not let your fingers touch the wound. As soon as possible cover the wound as follows:

Lay several thicknesses of sterile gauze over the wound. Cover this with a layer of absorbent cotton, and bind the whole with the triangular bandage or with the ribbon roller bandage. (See Bandaging, pages 36-50.)

No one but a physician should ever attempt to stitch a wound.

In most cases, the parts may be drawn together with the ribbon bandage, and over this the dressings applied.

Adhesive plaster should not be applied directly to a wound. It may be used over the bandage to hold it in place.

Do not bandage a wound too tightly unless it is necessary to stop bleeding.

After bandaging, keep the injured part in a position of comfort.

If the head is injured, make the patient lie down with his head resting upon a pillow or cushion covered with a clean towel.

If the forearm is injured, bring it across in front of the chest and support it in a sling.

If the leg be wounded, it may be supported upon a cushion or blanket.

In wounds of the chest raise the head and shoulders until the patient is able to breathe comfortably.

If the abdomen be wounded, place the patient on his back, with his knees drawn up. If the abdomen is cut from right to left, bend the head and chest forward to keep the wound closed. Watch for shock. Dress as for an ordinary wound.

In all cases watch for fracture and handle carefully.

Lacerated Wounds—These are quite common in industrial accidents. They are also caused by missiles, such as stones, or bricks, or by falling upon sharp stones and broken glass.

In cases of this sort, bleeding is not usually excessive. When the services of a physician cannot be secured, cover the wound immediately with clean dressings. Then place the patient in a comfortable position to await the arrival of a physician or transportation.

Pierced or Punctured Wounds—These are caused in war by bayonets, swords and similar weapons, and in civil life by needles, thorns, fishhooks, bits of glass, splinters, and other articles.

The simplest treatment is the best. Unless an object like a needle can be easily removed leave it until the arrival of a physician. In pulling out the needle or other object, use a pincers or tweezer that has just been boiled in water. Examine the object to see if it is complete. If any portion of it has been left in the wound, do not try to remove it, but inform the physician.

All objects which penetrate the flesh may carry infection into the wound. Swab with iodine or mercurochrome. Cover with sterile gauze and bind with a bandage.

To remove a splinter or other object imbedded in the flesh, take an ordinary penknife, pass the blade once or twice through the flame of a lamp (a large needle may also be used). Cover the fingers with sterile gauze. Slip the point of the penknife under the end of the splinter or other object, and catch it against the blade with the thumb and nail and draw it out. (Fig. 22.)

Do not attempt to remove objects imbedded in the flesh of the eye. Do not apply iodine to the eye.

Fishhooks and barbed points usually do not penetrate deeply and should be pushed through the tissues, never drawn back unless the barbed point has been cut off.

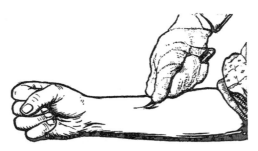

Fig. 22—Method of removing a splinter, using a knife blade. Fingers covered with gauze.

Gunshot wounds should be treated like other wounds. First check the bleeding, if it is severe, and make the patient as comfortable as possible. Swab the wound with iodine or mercurochrome and cover with a bandage. Watch for shock.

Bruises—To slight bruises apply lint or surgically clean plain gauze, folded and dipped in water. Apply cold water to severe bruises.

In cases involving shock, apply warm blankets, hot bottles, hot flat-irons covered with cloth, in fact, anything hot or warm, covered so as not to burn the skin. Give hot drinks, preferably coffee. Do not give alcoholic drinks.

POISONED WOUNDS

Snake Bite—Don't stop to kill the snake. Tear open the clothing to expose the wound quickly. Apply pressure with the thumb and finger, encircling the limb between the bite and the heart. Put a handkerchief, strap, rope, belt or suspender around the limb above the wound. Draw it just tight enough to check circulation.

Lay open the one or two holes made by the snake's fangs with the tip of a knife blade. Pass the blade down into the wound and cut outward about one inch—cut lengthwise rather than around the limb. Be careful not to cut an artery, but if severe bleeding occurs, stop it by pressure. Make the blood run from the knife cut. Rub the wound with the finger to dislodge any of the tenacious poison which remains. An oft-practiced and successful plan is to suck the wound, to extract the poison; there is no danger from the poison taken into the mouth, provided there are no cracks in the lip or badly decayed teeth, but it must not be swallowed. Encourage the wound to bleed by bathing in warm (not hot) water. Wash the wound with whisky if you wish, but do not give whisky to the sufferer.

Take the patient to a physician as soon as possible.

If a physician cannot be procured, wash the wound with water, or if possible to secure the material, fill the wound with common baking soda or permanganate of potash moistened with water. The wound may be swabbed with solution of iodine if at hand.

Release the pressure bandage every twenty minutes while you count three and then re-tighten.

Anti-Snake Bite Serum—One of the remarkable advances in the treatment of snake bite has been the perfection of Anti-Venom or Anti-Snake Bite Serum. This serum is an effectual antidote against the poison of the rattlesnake, the copper-head and the moccasin.

This serum is to be injected into the wound as soon as possible after the infection of the bite, but it will act if applied within twelve to twenty-four hours after the victim has been bitten.

The serum may be used by a layman, and even by the victim himself, if a doctor is not available.

The serum is supplied for use in a convenient syringe, with a needle attached, ready for immediate administration.

In snake bite cases when it is necessary to wait for the application of the serum, the methods of treatment here outlined should be followed, such as the opening of the wound, the application of pressure to prevent the spreading of the poison, the application of permanganate of potash, etc. The serum treatment to follow as soon as available.

Anti-Venom Serum should be kept at hand in lumber and other camps, and it should be carried by hunters, vacationists, and others where there is a possibility of exposure to snake bites.

The serum will keep unchanged for several years.

Anti-Venom Serum may be considered as an insurance against the effects of a poisonous snake bite.

The serum may be obtained through drug stores and dealers in medical supplies.

Bites of Dogs—Make the wound bleed freely. Apply solution of iodine to wound.

Do not kill the dog, but confine him so he cannot bite others. Wait to learn if he has rabies.

Cases of hydrophobia are serious. In all cases of dog bite, summon a physician and take his advice.

Bites of rats, cats and other animals are less dangerous than those of dogs. Apply tincture of iodine. Summon a physician.

Stings of Scorpions, Centipedes, Tarantulas —Apply ammonia at the point where the sting entered, then apply cold water or ice and summon a physician.

As a rule, a stinging insect leaves its sting in the wound. This should be forced out, if possible, by pressing on the skin at its side with a knife blade.

The stings of ordinary insects, such as spiders, mosquitoes, etc., should be wet with a solution of table salt or ammonia, then covered with baking soda or clay, and bandaged. Cold water may also be applied.

FRACTURES—BROKEN BONES

Simple Fracture—A break of the bone without a wound or injury of surrounding flesh.

Compound Fracture—A break of the bone where there is a wound or opening through the flesh to the fracture.

Send for a physician in all cases.

An invariable rule should be not to move the patient until the fractured part is supported by a splint—"splint where they lie."

Place the patient in as comfortable a position as possible, supporting the injured portion upon a pillow, a cushion or a pad of cloth or other material. All fractures should be supported from underneath, one hand above and one below the fracture.

If clothing is to be taken off, remove it from the sound part first, being careful to avoid giving pain to the patient by unnecessary handling. Cut the clothing in the seams, if possible.

Handle a fractured limb as carefully as you would a piece of rare china. Do not attempt to set the bone.

First aid workers should learn, under the guidance of a physician, how to apply a gentle traction while handling a fractured part. In fractures where a bone is protruding, do not use traction.

In all fractures when a physician cannot be obtained, support the fractured limb, at the spot where found, if possible. When it is necessary to move the patient, lay the limb upon a cushioned splint, and apply a bandage to keep the parts quiet and in such a way as to prevent the fragments of bones moving upon one another.

In compound fractures, before applying the splints, treat the bleeding, swab with a solution of iodine or mercurochrome and cover the wounds with sterile gauze, padded with absorbent cotton, and wrapped with a triangular bandage. Apply a splint as in a simple fracture, being careful not to bandage too tightly.

Splints—Use the chest as a splint for the arm by fastening the arm to the side with a wide roller bandage or with the triangular bandage, place a small pad between the arm and the body.

The uninjured leg will make a good temporary splint for a broken leg. In order to support a broken limb properly, the splint must extend above and below the injury so as to keep the joints and fragments quiet. The width of a splint should be a little greater than the thickness of the injured limb. Cushion the surface of the splint which is to come next to the limb with some soft and elastic materials or with ordinary cotton. Roller bandages should not be applied beneath the splint.

In many cases it is better to have two splints, one on each side of the limb, both held in place by the same bandage. Small splints may be cut from cigar boxes, pasteboard boxes, book covers, laths, shingles, flour or sugar barrel staves, broom or mop handles. Even fire-tongs, pokers, shovels and desk rulers have been employed. Cover well with soft paper, or absorbent cotton, lint, or gauze.

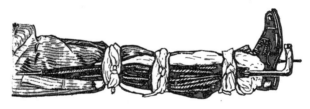

Fig. 23—Splint made with umbrella.

In the shop or factory, tools and their handles, umbrellas, canes or parasols, may be used. (Fig. 23.) In the absence of these, bunches of twigs from bushes, heavy folds of paper, straw or stiff grass may be utilized. In the army, soldiers utilize bayonets, swords, ramrods, rifles, and other articles for temporary splints.

Apply the triangular bandage folded as a broad or narrow cravat, or a roller cotton bandage, to hold the splints in place. If these are lacking, pocket handkerchiefs, towels, garters, suspenders, cords or straps may be used.

In applying a splint, the help of a second person should be obtained to support the limb while the dressings are being adjusted. In fixing a splint, avoid causing pain or bandaging the part so tightly as to interfere with the circulation of the blood. In raising a broken limb, support it above, underneath and below the injury, so that there is no bending of the limb at the point of injury. Bending causes pain and tearing of the soft parts.

In applying splints to the upper part of the body, let the patient be seated on a chair, the assistant, if there is one, working from behind the patient.

When it is necessary to move the patient, lay the limb, if it be the lower leg, upon a wooden support.

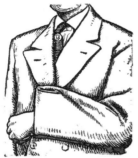

Fig. 24—Sling made with the sleeve of a coat.

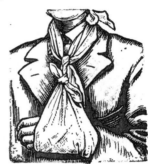

Fig. 25—Sling made with two handkerchiefs.

Slings—The triangular bandage or roller bandage can easily be made into a sling to support a broken limb. (See Bandaging.)

When bandages are lacking, utilize the sleeve as a sling for the arm by pinning it to the breast of the coat. (Fig. 24.)

Two handkerchiefs form an excellent sling. The first should be tied around the neck as loosely as possible, the second tied about the first in the same manner, and the arm slipped through it. (Fig. 25.)

Fracture of the Skull—Send immediately for a physician. Place the patient in a convenient shady place on his back with his head and shoulders slightly raised, the head lying on one side if the fracture is at the base.

Convey to a hospital as soon as possible.

If there is an open wound lay a pad or compress of sterile gauze and bandage very loosely over the wound.

{ 27 }

Fracture of the Nose—Apply cold and send the patient to a physician.

Fracture of the Jaw—Raise lower teeth to upper. Look for and remove false teeth. Apply bandages as illustrated, (Figs. 74-75), or use a cravat bandage.

Fracture of the Collar Bone—In fractures of the collar bone, the affected shoulder drops. The injured person usually supports the elbow and forearm with his free hand, so as to relieve the weight of the limb from the broken bone. Lay the patient on his back on a hard surface with a folded blanket under injured shoulder, without any pillow, until the physician arrives.

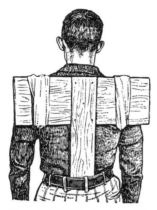

Fig. 26—Splint for fracture of the clavicle made of boards in cross form and bound over clothing. Useful when necessary to transport patient.

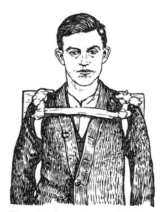

Fig. 27—Cross form splint for fractured clavicle. Front view.

Cover any wound present with gauze, loosely held in place. Before moving the patient, place a moderate sized pad of gauze, a cap, or soft cloth, in the armpit and bandage the arm to the chest. Let the forearm hang in a sling. The **T** shaped splint (**Figs. 26 and 27**) will form an excellent support and can be readily made from boards.

Fracture of the Spine—Send for a physician at once. Lay

the patient flat on his back. Do not disturb him unless absolutely necessary. Moving him may prove fatal. If necessary to move, raise him carefully without bending the spine and slide a board splint beneath him. Turning a patient in this condition to one side, or on his face, may prove fatal. Apply hot blankets to the body to keep patient warm.

Fracture of the Shoulder Blade—Bandage the arm to the side as in a fracture of the collar bone.

Protect any bruises with sterile gauze and a bandage.

Fracture of the Ribs—Move the patient as little as possible. Raise his head and chest to make breathing easier. He may lie upon the uninjured side or on his back, or may stand up.

Apply a wide roller cotton bandage carried around the chest several times, or several triangular bandages placed so as to extend several inches below or above the injury. Before bandaging gently press the palm of the hand on the chest wall. If this affords relief, bandaging will do good; if painful, bandaging must be omitted. If the patient is coughing up blood, do not bandage.

Before applying the first bandage, have the patient, with arms raised above his head, take in a deep breath and then let it out (exhale) so as to almost empty the lungs. Bandage the chest while it is deflated.

Broken Thigh—Send for a physician at once. Lay the patient on his back, or a little inclined toward the injured side. Raise the head and shoulders slightly. Gently draw the leg out straight by exerted traction, keeping the toes pointed upward. Hold the foot until the two legs are tied together.

Cover any wound with sterile gauze. Prevent movement of the fractured bone. Apply a splint, using a board, broom handle, rifle or other rigid object that will extend from below the foot to the armpit. Pad the splint. Fasten the splint by bandages above and below the break, about the knee and ankle and one about the waist. Do not bandage over the stomach. Apply an inner splint also from the crotch to foot, or in its absence bandage the injured limb to the sound one.

Fracture or Cut of the Knee-Cap—Do not bend the leg. Place the patient on his back with the injured leg somewhat elevated upon pillows. Cover any wound with sterile gauze. Make a pad about three inches thick out of paper or a towel wrapped in sterile gauze or lint. Place this pad in the hollow at the bend of the knee. Place a similar pad on the under part of the heel. Prepare a splint long enough to reach from below the heel to the middle of the thigh under the leg. Bind the splint at the ankle and the thigh, and also above and below the knee. (Fig. 29.)

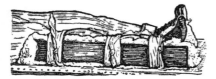

Fig. 28—Splint made of padded boards.

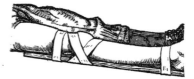

Fig. 29—Splint for fracture of knee-pan: may be fastened with adhesive plaster or bandages.

Fracture of the Leg Below the Knee—Lay the patient on his back. Draw the leg down straight and place it on a soft pillow or cushion, with the toes pointing upward.

Cover any wound with sterile gauze. Place a padded splint made of boards or sticks on each side of the leg, extending from the ankle joint to middle of thigh and bandage firmly. If a splint is not at hand, use a pillow, or many layers of paper. (Fig. 28.)

Broken Joints—Breaks near the joints are very serious and need extreme care. Bend or move the joint as little as possible. Apply light splints on all sides of the joints.

Lay the limb on a pillow.

Fracture of the Foot—Make a right-angle splint (Fig. 30), padded well with cotton or lint, and bandage to the side of the foot. Bandage another splint on the sole of the foot.

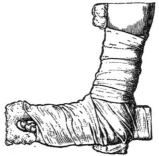

Fig. 30—Splint for foot made of two pieces of board.

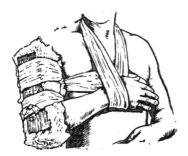

Fig. 31—Splint and bandage for fracture of upper arm.

Broken Upper Arm—Place a pad of folded cloth in the armpit extending under the arm from crotch to elbow. Draw the elbow down to the side. Bind the upper arm to the side of the chest with the triangular, or wide ribbon bandage. Place the forearm in a sling, so arranged that the hand is slightly higher than the forearm. For a fracture in the middle of the upper arm apply narrow splints on two sides of the arm. Secure by roller bandage and place the forearm in a sling. (Fig. 31.)

Fracture of the Forearm—Place the forearm across the chest, the palm of the hand turned in and the thumb pointing upward. Place padded splints on the outer and inner sides of arm from the elbow to below the wrist. (Fig. 32.) Bandage the splints and place the arm in a sling.

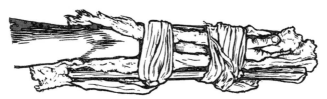

Fig. 32—Splint for fracture of forearm.

Fracture of the Wrist—Apply a well padded splint made of pieces of wood, cigar boxes, pasteboard, tin, wire or other material. The pad should extend from the finger tips well up to the forearm on the inner side of the hand. Place a similar pad upon the back of the hand and wrap the whole wrist smoothly in a bandage before applying the splint. Hang in triangular bandage sling.

Fracture of the Hand—Make a splint from thin wood, cigar boxes, pasteboard or any stiff material, long enough to extend from the finger tips to the middle of the forearm. Pad this splint

{ 31 }

well and apply it to the palm, taking care to have a thick wad of padding in the palm.

Bind the splint in place with bandages, and put the arm in a sling, with the hand slightly higher than the elbow.

Fracture of the Fingers—Make a splint of cardboard or any suitable material, sufficiently long to extend from the tip of the finger up to the wrist. Pad the splint with cotton and bind it firmly in place. Support the hand with a small sling.

Suggestions on Fractures

Treat all fractures with great care. In doubtful cases treat as a fracture.

In fractures it is all important to prevent further damage. Secure medical aid, provide proper transportation of the patient. Apply splints on the spot.

Do not attempt to handle the patient until splints have been applied.

If skull, spine, pelvis or lower limbs are broken, keep patient lying down.

Control bleeding if present before the applying of splints.

In broken joints splints must extend above and below the fracture.

When possible, splint arm to trunk, leg to leg, and lower joint to upper.

Look out for a shock.

Keep the patient warm so as to lessen the effects of shock.

Apply splints before attempting to move the patient.

BURNS AND SCALDS

THREE degrees are generally recognized:
Simple reddening of the skin—first degree.

The formation of blisters—second degree.

Charring of the skin, up to complete destruction of the part—third degree.

In all burns, send for a physician.

Burns of the second and third degree require immediate medical attendance. In severe burns there is liability of shock and prostration.

Shock should be treated before giving attention to the burn.

When a person's clothing catches fire, make him lie down. Throw him down if necessary. Wrap him quickly in a blanket, cloak, or shawl, preferably some woolen material, and smother the fire by pressing and slapping upon the burning points from the outside, beginning at the head, and then dash on water.

After placing the patient in a place of safety, remove clothing. If the clothing sticks, do not pull it off, cut around it and leave it for the physician to remove.

Burns are intensely painful. Contact with air increases the pain. Expose only small areas at a time and dress them promptly so as to exclude the air.

Do not expose the burn to heat, though warm, moist cloths are sometimes helpful, especially if wet with a warm solution of baking soda.

If a physician cannot be had at once, any of the methods here noted may be followed. In shops where burns are of frequent occurrence and even in households, materials suitable for application to burns should be kept at hand.

In cases of severe shock it is heroic but satisfactory treatment, when possible, to lay the patient on a sheet and lower him, clothes and all, into a bath tub of moderately warm water. This will relieve the pain and shock.

Cover slightly burned or scalded places with pieces of lint or gauze dipped in baking soda solution (one teaspoonful baking soda to one pint boiled water); cover this with absorbent cotton and finally wrap with the triangular or roller bandage.

In more severe cases, saturate a gauze pad with olive oil, sweet oil, vaseline or petrolatum. Carron oil (equal parts of raw linseed oil and lime water), while old-fashioned, is useful for emergency treatment. Lacking oils, dust the burned part with baking powder or boracic acid. Cover the whole area with a layer of lint, or gauze, and finally wrap with a triangular bandage.

A dressing for burns of all classes which is in accredited use is picric acid gauze. Picric acid gauze should not be used with ointments. It should always be moistened before applying.

Many first aid outfits contain a burn dressing ointment containing three per cent of bicarbonate of soda in petrolatum.

A weak solution of tannic acid applied on gauze or lint is a dressing used in many shops.

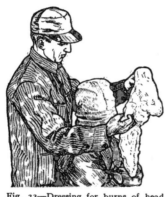

Fig. 33—Dressing for burns of head, neck, ears and face, made with picric acid gauze and covered with cotton.

Burns from caustic lye, strong ammonia and similar substances should first be flooded thoroughly with water and then treated as if caused by fire.

Burns from acid, vitriol and similar fluids should first be flooded with water. After washing, treat as a burn by fire.

Burns from carbolic acid are relieved if quickly washed with full strength grain alcohol.

If acids get into the eye, flush the eye with plenty of water. Cream or boracic acid solution may be used after washing.

In the case of burning of the lips and mouth by an acid use the same method.

Burns of the inside of the mouth or throat are caused by drinking hot fluids or swallowing chemicals. Apply olive oil or the white of an egg, by making the patient drink it or by pouring it from a spoon into the throat. In the case of burns by caustic potash, ammonia and the like, flush the mouth and throat with plenty of water and weak vinegar.

In case of scalding of the mouth and throat by steam, sometimes happening to children, wrap the patient in a blanket, summon a physician, apply hot flannels to the throat. Administer small doses of equal parts of olive oil and lime water.

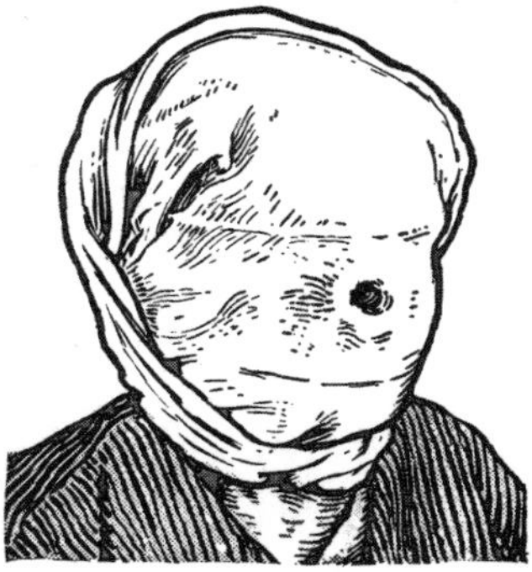

If a fragment of lime gets into the eye, do not try to take out the lime, but flush the eye freely with water. Castor oil may be dropped into the eye if a physician will not arrive soon.

Burns from gunpowder are to be treated in the same way as ordinary burns.

Fig. 34—Completed dressing of burns as shown in Fig. 33. Two triangular bandages used, with the base around the neck; one at the front and the second at the back and the ends tied around the neck and points tucked in.

Burns by electricity or lightning are to be treated in the same way as burns by fire.

Sun Burns—Treat as a mild scald, covering with a weak solution of baking soda, oils, vaseline, cold cream, then bandage.

FIRST AID BANDAGING

Two kinds of bandages are available for first aid work. They are known as the roller bandage and the triangular or handkerchief bandage. Both of these may be purchased at drug stores, or in an emergency they may be made on the spot. The roller bandages as purchased are made of surgical gauze or of muslin.

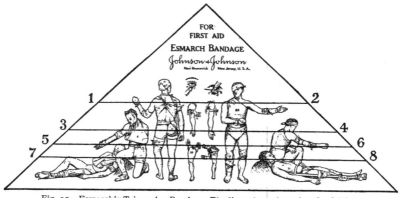

Fig. 35—Esmarch's Triangular Bandage. The lines show the points for folding.

The roller bandages made of surgical gauze are absorbent, thin and very pliable. They are suitable for placing next to a wound, or as agents for the application of fluid to the part. Cotton or muslin roller bandages are much stronger than those which are made of gauze, and are, therefore, more suitable where pressure or support is desired.

Except in great urgency, bandages should not be improvised, as the material usually at hand cannot be made to take the place of clean material, prepared especially for surgical uses.

Only when it is absolutely necessary should bandages be pieced, as pieced bandages are rough and may exert undue pressure upon the parts treated.

THE TRIANGULAR BANDAGE

THE Triangular or Esmarch Bandage is made by cutting a piece of cloth thirty-six or forty inches square into two pieces diagonally. Such a bandage can easily be improvised, but is obtainable from druggists. The triangular bandage has proven of the greatest value in emergencies, upon the field of battle and elsewhere. It is simple, efficient and of wide usage. It is probable that no other article used in wound dressing can accomplish so much, and in such a reliable manner, as this triangular bandage in rendering first aid.

Triangular bandages carrying the illustrations shown in Fig. 35 printed on the bandage can be purchased. It is recommended that first aid workers obtain one of these illustrated triangular bandages and familiarize themselves with its use. This can best be done by actual application of the bandage itself.

The triangular bandage is susceptible of many applications not shown in the illustrations. These will suggest themselves to the user. The bandage may be used either as a "broad" or "narrow" bandage.

The broad is made by spreading the bandage out, then bringing the point down to the lower border, and folding once.

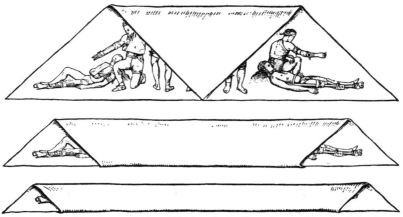

Fig. 36—Showing points at which to fold triangular bandage. For broad bandage bring the point over to the edge and fold once. For a narrow bandage bring the point to the edge and fold twice.

The narrow is made by drawing the point down to the lower border, and then folding twice. (See illustrations).

For the forehead, side of head, eye, cheek or any round part of the body (as the arm or thigh) the narrow bandage must be used, its center being placed on the wound, and the ends carried around and tied.

The bandage should always be fastened either with a pin or by a reef-knot or square knot (Figs. 40 and 41.) The so-called granny-knot should never be used. The triangular bandage may be applied to the body as follows:

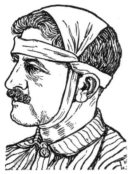 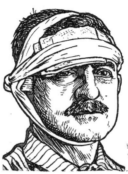 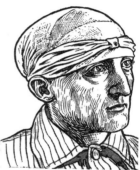

Fig. 37—Folded triangular bandage to apply pressure to the top of the head.

Fig. 38—Triangular bandage for the scalp.

Fig. 39 — Folded triangular bandage to apply pressure on artery and to hold pad in place on forehead. Useful in bleeding, etc.

To the Scalp (Fig. 37)—Fold a hem about two inches deep along the lower border. Place bandage on the head so that the hem lies on the forehead just above the eyebrows with the point

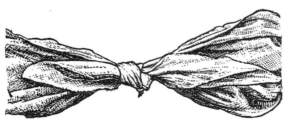 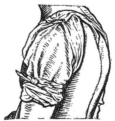

Fig. 40—Ends of triangular bandage tied into a reef-knot.

Fig. 41—Reef-knot.

drawn over the forehead. Then carry the two ends around the head above the ears, and tie in a reef-knot on the forehead. The point can then be drawn up and pinned at the top of the head. (See Figs. 37, 38, 39.)

For the eyes or front of the face the narrow bandage is folded about the head at the middle line of the face with the ends tied in a reef-knot.

For the Neck—Use the narrow or broad bandage as may be required, tying on the side opposite the injury. (See Figs. 42 and 43.)

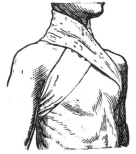
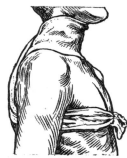
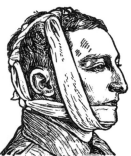

Fig. 42—Triangular bandage for back of neck.

Fig. 43—Triangular bandage for the neck.

Fig. 44—Triangular bandage for fracture of jaw, using two bandages folded very narrow.

For the Shoulder—Place the center of the bandage on the injured shoulder, with the point running up the side of the neck.

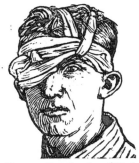
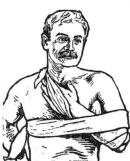
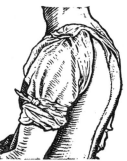

Fig. 45—Eye dressing; folded triangular bandage, gauze pad and roller bandage.

Fig. 46—Dressing for fracture of left collar bone—pad in armpit, two triangular bandages.

Fig. 47—Shoulder dressing held in place by triangular bandage.

Carry the ends around the middle of the arm and return and tie them on outside. Take a second bandage, fold it into a broad bandage, place one end over the point of the first bandage, and make a sling for the arm by carrying the other end of the bandage over the sound shoulder, and tying at the side of the neck. Bring the point of the first bandage under the part of the sling resting on the injured shoulder, draw it tight, turn it down and pin it.

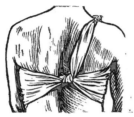 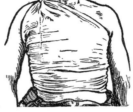 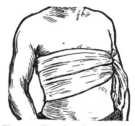

Fig. 48—Triangular bandage applied to chest. Back view. Fig. 49—Triangular bandage applied to chest. Front view. Fig. 50—Dressing for fracture of ribs—two triangular bandages with pad under the knot.

For the Chest (Figs. 48 and 49.) Place the middle of the bandage on the injured side, with the point over the shoulder. Carry the two ends around the waist and tie them. Then draw the point over the shoulder and tie to one of the ends, or extend with a piece of roller bandage.

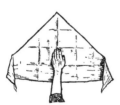 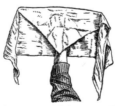 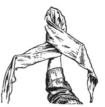

Fig. 51 — Triangular bandage dressing for hand. First move. Fig. 52 — Triangular bandage for hand. Second move. Fig. 53 — Triangular bandage for hand. Third move. Fig. 54 — Triangular bandage for hand. Completed bandage.

For the Back—The bandage is applied as above, but its application is begun by placing it on the back.

In injury to the ribs it is best to use two broad bandages,

applying one well under the armpits and the other one directly below, tying each at a point opposite the injury.

For the Forearm and Wrist—Bind with a broad cravat bandage and support the arm in a sling.

For the Hand—To cover the whole hand, the triangular bandage is spread out and the hand laid upon it with the wrist

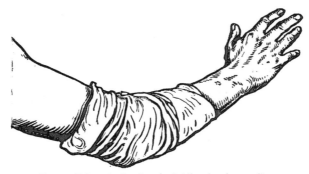

Fig. 55—Triangular bandage for holding dressing on elbow.

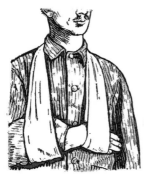

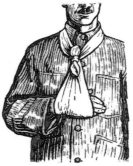

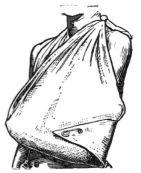

Fig. 56—Sling made of two triangular bandages. Tie ends together and place around the neck so as to make two loops.

Fig. 57—Sling made of triangular bandages, or two handkerchiefs.

Fig. 58—Triangular bandage broad sling for left arm.

at the lower border and the fingers toward the point. The point is carried back toward the fingers. The ends are brought about the wrist, crossed, brought back and tied. (Figs. 51 to 54.) This makes a very effectual and complete bandage for the whole hand and a support for all the fingers.

Large Arm Sling(Fig. 58.) —Spread out a bandage, put one end over the shoulder of the uninjured side and let the other hang down in front of the chest. Carry the point behind the elbow of the injured arm, and bend the arm forward over the middle of the bandage. Then carry the second end over the shoulder of the injured side, and tie it to the other end. Bring the point forward and pin it to the front of the bandage.

Small Arm Sling—Two triangular bandages are folded into the broad form, the ends tied together and placed around the

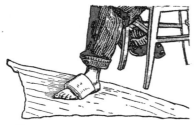

Fig. 59—Triangular bandage applied to foot to hold dressing in place.

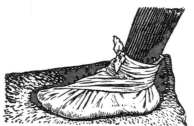

Fig. 61—Triangular bandage applied o foot.

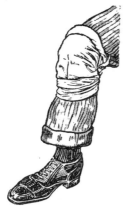

Fig. 62—Triangular bandage applied to knee.

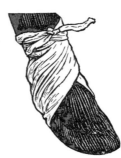

Fig. 60—Triangular bandage applied to heel.

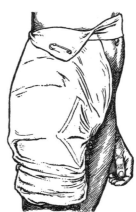

Fig. 63—Triangular bandage for the hip.

neck in such a way as to make two loops; one loop supports the forearm, and the other the hand. (Fig. 56.) A wider sling, consisting of one loop, is made of triangular bandages or two handkerchiefs. (Fig. 57.)

For the Hip (Fig. 63.)—Pass a narrow bandage around the body above the hip bones, tying the knot on the same side as the injury. Take another bandage, turn up a hem according to the size of the patient, place its center on the wound, carry the ends around the thigh, and tie them. Then carry the point up under the waist-band, turn it down over the knot, and pin it.

For the Foot—Spread out a bandage, place the foot on its center with the toe toward the point, draw up the point over the instep, bring the two ends forward, cross, and tie them around the ankle. (Figs. 59-6c-61.)

For the thigh, knee and leg, the cravat bandage may be used as shown in the illustrations.

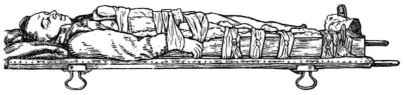

Fig 64—Dressing for fracture of thigh made with triangular bandages and padded splints. Sling made by tying ends of bandages together.

THE ROLLER BANDAGE

Roller bandages as supplied by druggists are made of muslin cloth, known as Cotton Roller Bandages, and of surgical gauze cloth, known as Gauze Bandages. Such bandages can be procured in widths of 1, 1½, 2, 2½, 3, 3½ and 4 inches. Roller bandages made of gauze are supplied in ten-yard lengths. The cotton roller bandages are supplied in five-yard lengths.

The roller bandage is easily applied, and while experience is necessary, with a little practice any layman may make an application that will answer in an emergency.

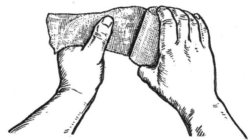

Fig. 65—Method of handling roller bandage.

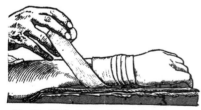

Fig. 66—Method of applying roller bandage spirally, beginning with slow spiral turns.

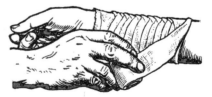

Fig. 67—Method of reversing or folding back turns of the spiral roller bandage.

It is not to be expected that the untrained layman will apply a bandage as correctly as would a physician. The important point in the application of a bandage is to cover the injury, hold dressings or splints in place, until the patient is turned over to the care of a physician.

Trained workers in first aid may practice under a physician,

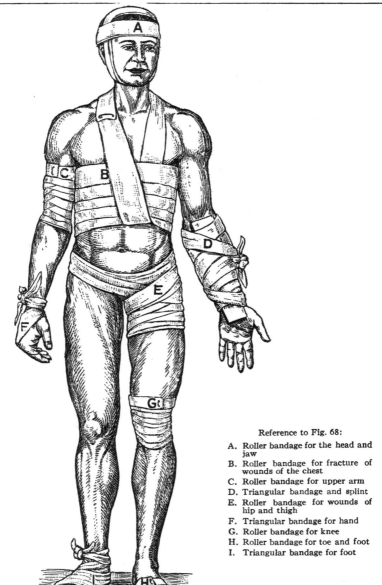

Reference to Fig. 68:

A. Roller bandage for the head and jaw
B. Roller bandage for fracture of wounds of the chest
C. Roller bandage for upper arm
D. Triangular bandage and splint
E. Roller bandage for wounds of hip and thigh
F. Triangular bandage for hand
G. Roller bandage for knee
H. Roller bandage for toe and foot
I. Triangular bandage for foot

Fig. 68—Method of applying Triangular and Roller Bandages.

consult the illustrations here shown, and thus, by practice, acquire skill in bandaging.

To apply a roller bandage, begin by holding the extremity at the point at which it is to start with the thumb and index finger of the left hand. Hold the roll of bandage in the right hand and turn this hand in the direction taken by the hands of a clock, unrolling the bandage and at the same time turning it around the part to be enclosed. Make the first turn with the right hand, after which the left hand, being freed by the overlapping, may alternate with it.

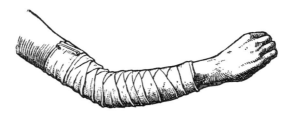

Fig. 69—Roller bandage for elbow joint; begin bandaging at forearm.

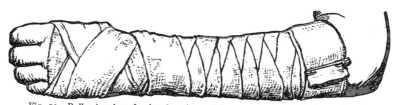

Fig. 70—Roller bandage for hand, wrist and forearm; begin bandaging at hand.

The simplest form of application of a roller bandage is a direct circular turn around the part beginning at the end of the limb or other part. Where the part is larger at one end than the other (for example, the forearm from the wrist to the elbow), circular turns do not lie smoothly. In such cases begin at the small end, making a few turns each over the other, and then move the turns up the limb spirally, making the spirals overlap each other about one-third their width.

When the bandage begins to pucker, turn the edge so as to make an inverted V and carry around the part overlapping the preceding turn, and so on, repeating the process until the whole part is covered. (Figs. 66 and 67.)

At the joints—elbow, knee, ankle—the roller bandage may be applied so as to form a figure 8, the bend of the joint forming the crossing part or middle of the figure 8, with loops above and below the joint. (Fig. 69.)

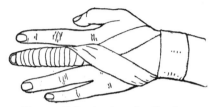

Fig. 71—Roller bandage for the finger; begin at the wrist.

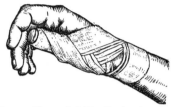

Fig. 72—Figure-of-eight roller bandage for the thumb; begin at the wrist.

In applying a roller bandage, care must be used as to the amount of tension to be employed. Surgeons use the expressions "tight," "moderately tight" and "loose." These degrees may be estimated by applying a bandage to one's own person. A tight bandage around the hand causes it to throb. A moderately tight bandage around the fingers gives the support of a

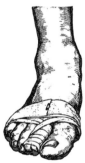

Fig. 73—Roller bandage for the toe; begin at the foot.

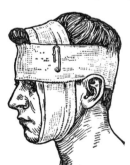

Fig. 74—Roller bandage for the head and jaw.

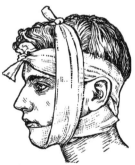

Fig. 75—Roller bandage for injuries of the chin.

comfortably fitting glove. A loose bandage is one that may be applied to the eye without discomfort. As a general rule, bandages around the fleshy part of the arm and the thigh may be applied with more force than those on other parts of the body. When the roller bandage is used to hold dressings or splints in place, more pressure may be used than if it is applied directly to the limb itself.

In bandaging the hand or foot, the tips of fingers or toes, with a roller bandage, the nails should be left uncovered unless they have been injured, in order to make sure circulation is not impeded. If the nails are bluish in color the bandage should be loosened.

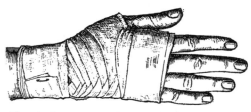

Fig. 76—Roller bandage for back of hand and wrist; begin at wrist.

The tip of the elbow or the heel should not be covered unless injured.

Bandages applied over thick layers of gauze or cotton can be made tighter than those applied where no other dressing is employed. It should also be noted that a limb bandaged when elevated, will, when lowered or extended, distend and increase the pressure. When

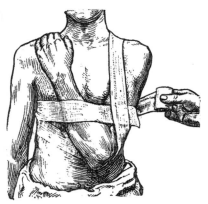

Fig. 77—Roller bandage for fracture of the shoulder. First step.

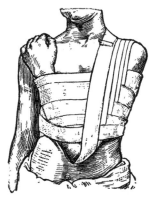

Fig. 78—Roller bandage for fracture of the shoulder. Finished bandage.

a bandage is started at the ankle and passed on to the extremity of the foot and then returned to the ankle, the first winding should be very loose. Allowance should be made in bandaging for any shrinkage which may occur as a result of the wetting of the bandage by discharge from the wounds or bleeding.

Aged persons and children should be bandaged only loosely.

In applying bandages to the chest, breathing should not be hindered.

To secure the end of a roller bandage, pins or strips of adhesive plaster may be used. The end of the bandage may be slit into tails, carried around the part in opposite directions and tied. If a pin is used, it should always be directed downwards and appear to view at least twice through the layers of cloth, its point being buried in the bandage.

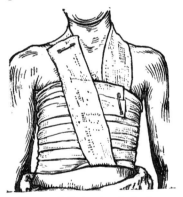

Fig. 79—Roller bandage for fracture of ribs or wounds of the chest.

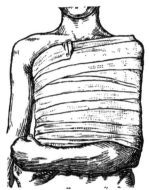

Fig. 80—Roller bandage for wounds of shoulder or armpit.

Sizes of Bandages

Roller bandages vary in width and length according to the use for which they may be desired. The following sizes are those most fre-quently used:

Bandages for the hand, fingers and toes—1 inch wide, 1 to 2 yar⌐ in length.

Bandages for the head, arms and legs of children—1½ or 2 inch wide, 6 yards in length.

Bandages for the arms, legs and extremities of adults—2½ incʰ wide, 6 to 8 yards in length.

Bandages for the thigh, groin and trunk—3 inches wide, 8 to yards in length.

Rules for Applying the Roller Bandage

Fix the bandage by taking one or two turns round the part.

Bandage from below upwards and from within outwards over the front of the limb.

The pressure must be equal throughout.

Each succeeding turn should overlap two-thirds of its predecessor.

Keep the margins parallel and all crosses and reverses in one line.

See that the part is in the position in which it is to remain after being bandaged.

When "reversing" make all the "reverses" downwards and on the outer side of a limb.

See that the bandage is tightly rolled up before commencing.

In taking off a bandage gather the slack in the hand.

End by fixing the bandage securely.

When Sending for a Doctor

When a person receives an injury and is thereby rendered unable to walk, considerable time elapses while he is being removed to his home. Much valuable time can, therefore, be saved by forwarding a message in advance to the doctor. It should contain details of the injury in the following order:

1. Part of the body injured: head, chest, abdomen, legs or arms.

. Right or left side, above or below knee or elbow.

Whether bleeding or not.

Conscious or unconscious.

Most particularly, correct name and address of person injured.

When possible to do so, send the message in writing.

SUNSTROKE AND HEAT PROSTRATION

SEND for a physician.

In sunstroke there is a slow and full pulse, labored breathing, a dry and hot skin, red face and unconsciousness. Remove the patient to a dry and shady place, loosening his collar, necktie, and any tight clothing. Raise the head and upper part of the body. Pour cold water over the head and face, and if very hot rub the body with pieces of ice. Use a fan freely. If removal to a hospital will be delayed, the patient may be placed in a tub of lukewarm water, the water gradually cooling.

In heat prostration there is a pale face, clammy skin, shallow breathing, weak and rapid pulse, sometimes there is unconsciousness. Place the patient flat on his back and loosen his clothing. Apply heat to the surface of the body and extremities. Bathe the face with warm water.

In exhaustion from heat, due to hard work and confinement in a close, hot atmosphere, cover the body with blankets and apply heat to the extremities.

In prostration from drinking too much ice water when overheated, loosen the patient's clothing, place him on his back with his head slightly elevated. Give hot drinks, apply heat to the spine and the extremities. Don't give alcoholic stimulants. Tea, coffee or warm milk may be used.

FROSTBITE

Carry the patient to a closed room without a fire and undress him carefully. Send for a physician.

Rub the frozen parts, or the whole body with snow or bits of ice. Give warm coffee or tea as a stimulant.

If the person has ceased breathing, use methods of artificial respiration. When the patient revives, carry him to a room slightly warmer, and cover loosely with a blanket.

Afterward rub with a cloth wet in warm water or diluted alcohol. Give beef tea, milk or ordinary tea as stimulants.

FAINTING

Fainting and shock resemble each other closely and are often confused. Shock usually follows severe injuries, is lasting and serious. Fainting is transitory. Shock is seldom accompanied by complete unconsciousness.

Fainting usually requires little treatment, unless the heart is diseased or very weak. Lay the fainting person out flat at once, with the head lower than the body. See that he has plenty of fresh air to breathe. Keep bystanders away.

Remove or loosen heavy wraps, tight collars, corsets and waistbands. Gently dab water upon the face, and hold smelling salts, spirit of camphor or ammonia under the nostrils, without touching them. Do not scald the nose of the patient by holding these applications too close or using them too long. Elevate and rub the limbs of the patient toward the body to quicken the circulation. If the person is slow in reviving, apply gentle heat, to the pit of the stomach. After recovery, give a cup of hot tea

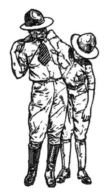

Fig. 81—Method of carrying a person who is fainting.

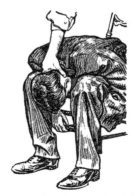

Fig. 82—Bending the head between the knees to prevent fainting.

or coffee, or a teaspoonful of aromatic spirit of ammonia in half a cup of water. Do not let the patient assume an erect position for some time after fainting. To prevent fainting bend the head between the knees (Fig. 82), but do not resort to this after fainting has taken place. Have the patient see a physician.

FITS—EPILEPSY

Treat fits in much the same way as fainting.

An epileptic should be laid upon his back with the head slightly raised. Loosen all tight clothing, remove all objects which might do harm if the limbs came against them. To prevent self-inflicted injury, the patient's arms and legs may be held gently but not pinned down, a folded towel or piece of soft wood between the teeth to prevent biting of the tongue.

When the convulsion has passed, allow the patient to sleep, and finally consult a physician.

Apoplectic strokes sometimes resemble epileptic fits. (See unconsciousness.)

If a patient suffers from hysteria, apply mustard plasters to the soles of the feet and to the wrists. Avoid dashing water in the face, or using strong emetics.

INSENSIBILITY—UNCONSCIOUSNESS

People are often found insensible by the roadside, on the street, and in other places; this condition may be due to several causes. It is often very difficult for an inexperienced first aid worker to distinguish between these varieties; such cases often perplex the experienced physician. However, it is safe for the worker to give first aid treatment along general lines as follows:

Send for medical assistance.

Place the patient in a position so as to insure easy breathing. When the patient's face is pale, keep the head low, on a line with the body; when the face is flushed, keep the head up.

When raising the head of an unconscious person, attention must be paid to maintaining a free passage of air through the windpipe; by raising the head, neck and shoulders together, so that the head is not bent sharply either forwards or backwards, the windpipe is kept quite straight.

Loosen all tight clothing.

Provide for a sufficiency of air. Keep the crowd at a distance; if indoors, open the doors and windows so that a free current of air is provided. Fanning will help to produce a circulation of air round the patient's head.

Allow an unconscious person to remain for a time where he lies, protecting him from rain or from the direct rays of the sun by holding an umbrella over him. When signs of consciousness return, he may be placed on a stretcher and carried to shelter. If, however, after a reasonable time (half hour, or more) unconsciousness still continues, removal becomes imperative without waiting for revival.

Examine for wounds, fractures and bleeding, and if necessary, care for these.

Give no stimulants or other liquids.

Observe and note the position of the body and whether the clothing is torn or disarranged, also the immediate surroundings.

Observe the state of the pupils, and the character of the breathing.

In aged persons, apoplexy may be suspected. In apoplexy, there is a flushed face and the pupils of the eyes are unequal in size. The face, on the injured side, has a squinty appearance, and the opposite side of the body is paralyzed. In apoplexy lay the patient on his back, head and shoulders raised, head to one side. Ice or cold water may be applied to the head, and warmth applied to the extremities. Do not move the patient until necessary to transport to a place of treatment.

Report your observations to the physician or other authorities.

If the person has to be removed, do so with caution. Take him to a hospital rather than to a police station.

SPRAINS AND STRAINS

Sprains may have serious results. Summon a physician at once, but start treatment pending his arrival.

In sprains there is a twisting and tearing of the ligaments at or near a joint, causing a rupture of the small blood vessels and bleeding under the skin. The swelling is caused by this bleeding and may be relieved by the application of cold, by pressure or proper placing.

Be on the watch for fractures, which at times resemble sprains. If in doubt, treat as fracture. Apply moist cold cloths. Immerse the foot in a bucket of cold water, adding more water, as cold as can be borne, for fifteen or twenty minutes. After this apply a firm bandage and elevate the foot. Repeat bathing treatment frequently.

Cold water applications may be continued by means of cloths dipped in very cold water, wrapped firmly around the part and frequently renewed.

Treat all sprains of joints in the same way.

Support a sprained arm or wrist always in a sling. Use a cushion or pad for a sprained foot or knee.

Place a sprained arm in a sling.

Give a sprained joint complete rest by using a splint and bandage.

Strains—A strain is a wrenching or tearing of muscle.

Apply a firm bandage or adhesive dressing over the injured part to keep the part at rest. It may be necessary to apply a splint. Do not apply iodine to a strain or sprain.

DISLOCATIONS

Send for the doctor at once. Do not attempt to treat a dislocation. Put the part in the position easiest to the sufferer, by using a sling for the arms and a cushion or other support for the legs, as in cases of fracture. If the pain is severe, apply either hot or cold wet cloths in the same manner as directed for sprains.

FOREIGN BODIES IN THE EYE, NOSE, EAR AND THROAT

Accidents of this character are complicated and at times very serious. Always send for a physician, and in the meantime carry out only such measures as will prevent further damage.

Foreign Substances in the Eye—Cinders, dust, sand and small objects can often be removed from the eye by simple means. Instruct the sufferer not to rub the eye, and to keep it closed. Tears will often wash such particles into the corners, where they can be seen and carefully removed with a wisp of absorbent cotton or surgical gauze.

If the body is lodged or hidden from view under the upper or lower lid, catch the upper lid by the lashes and pull it away from the eyeball and down over the lower lid; hold it there for a moment, then let the lid recede of itself. The free flow of tears may wash the dust particles into the corner of the eye, or they will be caught by the lower eyelid. Pulling down the lower eyelid will reveal the foreign body if it is lodged there.

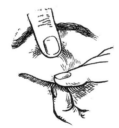 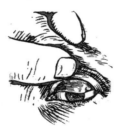 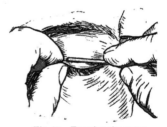

Fig. 83—Pulling the upper eyelid down to cause flow of tears.   Fig. 84—Everting the upper eyelid to locate foreign body in the eye.   Fig. 85—Everting the upper eyelid by pulling over a match.

Another way is to lift the upper lid and insert a clean piece of blotting paper between the lid and the eyeball. By removing the paper gently the foreign body may be caught and removed. Railroad men often carry strands of clean hair with them. (Sterile horse-hair can, by one who is practiced, be doubled and drawn between the eyeball and lid, and the foreign body dragged out.)

If these measures do not succeed, carefully inspect the mucous membrane and eyeball. Turn the upper lid. This is done as follows: The patient is told to look down, and while he does so, the edge of the upper lid is pulled first forward and downward by the lashes, then pulled away from the eyeball and upward over the point of the thumb or forefinger of the left hand, which is held on the lid. The lashes are then held against the edge of the eye socket. To assist in the examination a magnifying glass may be employed. (Figs. 83 and 84.)

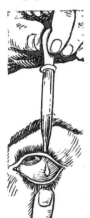

Remove any loose, visible foreign body with a bit of surgical gauze, or an absolutely clean piece of cloth or absorbent cotton, twisted with clean fingers around a match or toothpick.

Do not touch the eye with dirty fingers or with unclean cloth or pocket handkerchief.

Never use a knife blade, pencil or needle to remove particles of dust or cinders from the eye, or inflammation may set in and disastrous results follow.

If the fragment is imbedded in the eyeball, leave its treatment for a physician.

To allay any irritation after a substance is removed, wash the eye repeatedly with warm water containing a little salt (a small teaspoonful to the pint), or with a saturated boric acid solution, or put into the eye one or two drops of

Fig. 86—Dropping castor oil into the eye to allay irritation.

castor oil. Do not apply eye washes or poultices except under the direction of a physician.

Immediately after treatment cover the eye with surgical gauze, held in place by a roller or triangular bandage, loosely carried around the head. (See Bandaging.)

In all eye cases, no matter how trivial, have the sufferer see a physician.

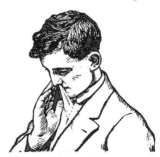

Fig. 87—Blowing the nose to remove foreign body.

Foreign Bodies in the Nose—Send for a physician. Have the patient blow his nose vigorously while holding the opposite nostril closed. Excite sneezing by tickling the nose or by snuffing pepper.

Foreign Bodies in the Ear—Unskilled efforts to remove foreign bodies in the ear are dangerous to the patient. Never insert wire, needles or pins into the ear to aid in removing bodies. The safest rule is to send the patient to a physician.

If live insects get into the ear, first pour into the ear-canal a little sweet oil or glycerin, then gently syringe it with warm water.

An ingenious method which is sometimes successful is to turn the ear at once toward a strong light and a living insect may come out of itself.

Foreign Bodies in the Throat—Summon a physician at once. Send him information as to the character of the accident, so that he may bring the needed instruments, as it may be necessary to open the throat to save life.

When there is no serious difficulty in breathing, delay all action until the doctor arrives.

To help the act of coughing, slap the person on the back while the patient's body is bent forward (face downward), and thus dislodge the bodies in the windpipe.

Facilitate the expulsion, if practical and possible, by lifting the person up by the heels so that the head hangs downward, and then slapping him on the back while in this position.

The patient may be tied to a bench with bandages, and then have his feet elevated by lifting the end of the bench.

If the substance can be seen, open the patient's mouth and press two fingers back into the throat so as to grasp it; even if the effort to grasp it is not successful, the act may produce vomiting, which may expel it.

After the foreign body has been extracted, if the person does not show signs of breathing, use artificial respiration.

ARTIFICIAL RESPIRATION

KNOWLEDGE of resuscitation by the application of artificial respiration is essential in every walk of life. Some of the cases requiring this form of aid may be summarized as follows:

Electrical shock where the body is stunned and breathing has stopped.

Asphyxiation, which arises when the body is deprived of air, as in the presence of illuminating gas, the gases of mines, gas from defective burning of stoves, exhaust gas from automobiles, ammonia fumes, gasoline fumes, gases from a blast furnace, gases from molten metals, vapors from bromine, chlorine, sulphur and formaldehyd, gases and fumes which arise in many chemical processes; exclusion of air, as in a closed vault; confined air, as in a ship's hold, cellars, old wells, etc.

Suffocation, which may follow the inhalation of sewer gas, smoke, etc.

Suspended breathing, which at times follows inhalation of chloroform, ether, over-doses of laudanum, and certain other drugs; stunning from falls, heavy blows, cave-ins, etc.

In these and emergencies of like type, the requirements for resuscitation are alike.

The supply of oxygen (air) is cut off in some cases by violence, in some cases by the substitution of noxious gases, and in others by failure to eliminate carbon dioxide produced in the tissue. But in all cases the breathing tissues are inhibited or paralyzed.

First aid treatment is an attempt to restore breathing, to induce air to enter the lungs, to do artificially what is done naturally in health.

This is performing artificial respiration.

Several methods of procedure have been used in the past, but in modern practice the Schaefer, or prone method, has been officially endorsed and generally adopted in this country.

In applying restoration methods, the first aid worker should ever have before him the following:

Send for a doctor, but while waiting, act promptly. A delay

of a moment may mean the loss of a life. Begin artificial respiration at once.

Avoid hurried or irregular motions. All methods depend for success upon the regularity and rhythm of the movements.

Avoid overcrowding, or an overheated room, giving stimulants before the patient can swallow, giving up too soon.

Do not use pulmotor or other apparatus except on specific direction of a physician.

SCHAEFER METHOD

This method, also known as the "prone" method, has been universally adopted as the standard method for producing artificial respiration.

The Schaefer method has the advantage of requiring but little muscular exertion, and for that reason it can be worked by one person alone.

Further advantages claimed for the prone-pressure method over other methods are: (1) Greater simplicity and ease of performance; (2) absence of trouble from the tongue falling back and blocking the air passages; (3) little danger of injuring the liver or breaking the ribs if pressure be gradually—not roughly—applied, and (4) larger ventilation of the lungs.

Schaefer or "prone" method of artificial respiration, as here given has been approved by:

> American Telephone & Telegraph Company
> American Red Cross
> American Gas Association
> Bethlehem Steel Company
> National Electric Light Association
> National Safety Council
> Bureau of Medicine & Surgery, Navy Department
> Office of the Surgeon-General, War Department
> U. S. Bureau of Mines
> U. S. Bureau of Standards
> U. S. Public Health Service and others

1. Lay the patient on his belly, one arm extended directly overhead, the other arm bent at elbow and with the face turned

{60}

outward and resting on hand or forearm so that the nose and mouth are free for breathing. (See Fig. 88.)

2. Kneel, straddling the patient's thighs with your knees placed at such a distance from the hip bones as will allow you to assume the position shown in Fig. 88.

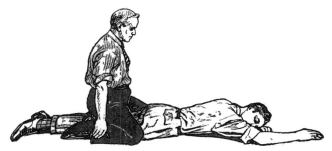

Fig. 88—Schaefer (or prone) method of artificial respiration. Position before beginning movements.

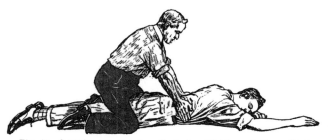

Fig. 89—Schaefer (or prone) method of artificial respiration. First movement.

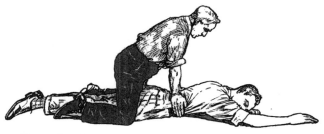

Fig. 90—Schaefer (or prone) method of artificial respiration. Second movement.

Place the palms of the hands on the small of the back with fingers resting on the ribs, the little finger just touching the lowest rib, with the thumb and fingers in a natural position, and the tips of the fingers just out of sight. (See Fig. 89.)

3. With arms held straight, swing forward slowly so that the weight of your body is gradually brought to bear upon the patient. The shoulder should be directly over the heel of the hand at the end of the forward swing. (See Fig. 90.) Do not bend your elbows. This operation should take about two seconds.

4. Now immediately swing backward so as to completely remove the pressure.

5. After two seconds, swing forward again. Repeat deliberately twelve to fifteen times a minute the double movement of compression and release, a complete respiration in four or five seconds.

6. Continue artificial respiration without interruption until natural breathing is restored, if necessary, four hours or longer, or until a physician declares the patient is dead.

7. As soon as this artificial respiration has been started and while it is being continued, an assistant should loosen any tight clothing about the patient's neck, chest, or waist. *Keep the patient warm.* Do not give any liquids whatever by mouth until the patient is fully conscious.

8. To avoid strain on the heart when the patient revives, he should be kept lying down and not allowed to stand up. If the doctor has not arrived by the time the patient has revived, he should be given some stimulant, such as one teaspoonful of aromatic spirit of ammonia in a small glass of water, or a hot drink of coffee, or tea, etc. The patient should be kept warm.

9. Resuscitation should be carried on at the nearest possible point to where the patient received his injuries. He should not be moved from this point until he is breathing normally of his own volition and then moved only in a lying position. Should it be necessary, due to extreme weather conditions, etc., to move the patient before he is breathing normally, resuscitation should be carried on during the time that he is being moved.

10. A brief return of natural respiration is not a certain indication for stopping the resuscitation. Not infrequently the patient after a temporary recovery of respiration, stops breathing again. The patient must be watched and if natural breathing stops, artificial respiration should be resumed at once.

11. In carrying out resuscitation, it may be necessary to change the operator. This change must be made without losing the rhythm of respiration. By this procedure no confusion results at the time of change of operator and a regular rhythm is kept up.

The above treatment should be persevered in for some hours, as it is an erroneous opinion that persons are irrecoverable because life does not soon make its appearance. Restoration has been accomplished after persevering for three to four hours.

The appearances which generally accompany death are:

Breathing and the heart's action cease entirely; the eyelids are generally half closed; the pupils dilated; the tongue approaches to the under edges of the lips, and these, as well as the nostrils, are covered with a frothy mucus. Coldness and pallor of surface increase.

Treatment After Breathing Has Been Restored

To promote warmth and circulation, commence rubbing the limbs upwards, with firm grasping pressure and energy, using handkerchiefs, flannels, etc. The friction must be continued under the blanket or over the dry clothing.

Promote the warmth of the body by the application of hot flannels, hot water bottles, heated bricks, etc., to the pit of the stomach, the arm-pits, between the thighs, and to soles of the feet.

If the patient has been carried to a house after respiration has been restored, be careful to let the air play freely through the room.

On the restoration of life, a teaspoonful of warm water should be given; and then, if the power of swallowing has returned, small quantities of aromatic ammonia, coffee or tea may be administered. Patient should be kept in bed, and a disposition to sleep encouraged.

Cautions

Prevent unnecessary crowding of persons round the body, especially if in an apartment.

Avoid rough usage, and do not allow the body to remain on the back unless the tongue is secured.

Under no circumstances hold the body up by the feet.

On no account place the body in a warm bath, unless under doctor's direction.

The method here outlined for artificial respiration is applicable in suspended breathing in cases of drowning, electric shock, accidents arising from illuminating gas, automobile exhaust gas, and suffocation from other causes.

How to Avoid Accidents

Look in the direction in which you are moving.

Always look both ways in crossing a street.

Never leave a car or other vehicle when it is in motion.

Never put your head or arms out of a moving vehicle.

Never play with firearms. Keep them beyond the reach of children.

Keep matches and medicines of all kinds out of the reach of children in your home.

Don't remain in a garage with the doors closed when the motor of the car is running.

Never allow a pin, needle or tack to drop to the floor without picking it up. It may mean lock-jaw for you or death for the child who may swallow it.

Do not use kerosene, benzine or other inflammable liquids in lighting a fire.

Never go out of a room and leave a lamp burning near a window curtain.

Never touch a wire which you find hanging in the street.

Do not take a lighted match into, or do not light a match in, a cellar, or anywhere that gas has escaped.

FIRST AID INSTRUCTION

THIS book is a working manual rather than a text-book. For this reason, as well as for the sake of conciseness, matters relating to the principles upon which the study and practice of first aid is founded, have been omitted.

Classes in first aid are now numerously organized in factories, mines, Y. M. C. A.'s, Boy Scout brigades, railway, police and fire departments, and in other institutions and associations.

From these a demand has been made for an outline system of instruction, with a manual as its basis. In response to this demand, and without attempting to give directions to instructors in first aid, the following suggestions are offered.

Classes in first aid may be formed wherever a teacher and one or two pupils can be brought together. Many hundred physicians throughout the country have voluntarily given their time to teaching first aid. Such self-sacrificing work is worthy of note, and should be appreciated.

If the services of a physician cannot be obtained, a trained nurse, a school teacher, a foreman or superintendent, can fit themselves for the task.

Pupils may come from any condition of life, and may be of either sex.

They should be persons of temperate habits. Persons who are alert, self-possessed and active are apt to make the greater progress.

Above all things, pupils should be selected from among those who enter into the work voluntarily, and who will industriously and conscientiously carry it on.

The lectures or talks may be given at intervals of about one week and should not exceed one hour in length. The pupils should be required to write out notes of the talks. The talks should be interspersed with or followed by demonstration and practice work.

The instructor should, in every lesson, strongly emphasize one point—the necessity of calling a physician in every emergency.

Pupils, above all things, should learn when to stop attempts at first aid, and place the patient in the hands of a physician.

In practice work, many instructors have found it convenient to use a Boy Scout, in tights and sweater, as a model. Instructors sometimes select two bright pupils from a class, and to these delegate the work of making the demonstration which in turn is followed by the class. When the pupils are girls the ordinary gymnasium suit will be found suitable for demonstration work.

Teaching and demonstration should be made with actual material.

Material used in practice work must not be used for wound dressing afterward, but should be kept apart for practice purposes.

A knowledge of anatomy and physiology is helpful, but not essential for efficient first aid work. There is a tendency on the part of instructors to pay too much attention to the details of anatomy and physiology. At best, these subjects are difficult and uninteresting.

Experienced teachers have found that the only knowledge of anatomy and physiology necessary is a full comprehension of the arterial and venous system, the location of the principal organs, and a general outline of the bony structure. This can be imparted by the aid of pictures or diagrams, coupled with demonstrations upon a model. This is about all that any ordinary class can absorb. The danger of infection of wounds is of prime importance, however, for consideration in the bandaging of injuries and the transportation of patients.

It is found that students make much greater progress when their studies are confined to acquiring ability to handle cases of injury and illness which they may encounter.

Instructors should select subjects with due consideration of the likeliest accidents in the work of the life of the local people. Accidents incident to sports are of particular interest to the younger generation.

The course of instruction may be preceded by a general talk on first aid, its nature, value and necessity in every walk of life.

A course of instruction in first aid may be made to cover a period varying from three months to two or more years. There is always something to learn.

In each succeeding lesson a review should be made of the previous topic, and at the close a review of all the topics should be given.

TOPIC I
The First Things to Do

(Manual references—pages 9 and 10)

The important points:

Keep cool. Summon a surgeon. Work quietly.
Place the patient in a comfortable position.
Remove clothing and ascertain nature of injury.
Stop bleeding, if present.
Dress wound if necessary.
Transport injured person to a place of safety.

Shock:

Its importance. Symptoms. Treatment—what to do and what not to do.

Demonstrations—Handling of patient, position, examination for injury, removal of clothing, methods of keeping warm, application of stimulants.

The important points of this lesson, so far as they relate to first things to do, should be continuously repeated.

TOPIC II
Bleeding

(Manual references—pages 11 to 18)

More than one lesson is required to completely cover this subject. It should arouse a discussion on the circulation of the blood.

Distinction between arterial, venous and capillary hemorrhage.

Location of main arteries of the body, with points where arterial circulation may be arrested with pressure. Pupils should locate these positions on their own body.

Dangers of hemorrhage.

Natural Arrest of Hemorrhage—Coagulation of the blood, contraction of blood vessels.

ʹ First aid in hemorrhage: direct pressure on bleeding part. Elevation of part. Application of cold. Pressure on arteries supplying wound.

Internal hemorrhage: spitting of blood, vomiting of blood, nose bleed.

Pupils should practice application of pressure to the arteries by hand, by the use of the tourniquet, and the compress.

They should improvise compresses, tourniquets and pads from objects ordinarily at hand in household or shop.

Caution pupils against touching the wound; against leaving a tourniquet on too long; against the use of stimulants in bleeding.

Calling a surgeon. Covering wounds.

TOPIC III

Wounds

(Manual references—Wounds, pages 19 to 24; bandaging, pages 36 to 50.)

This lesson and the three which follow involve the application of dressings and bandages.

The use of the Roller Bandage and the Triangular Bandage should be made the subject of special lessons or drills. The Triangular Bandage should be given precedence.

Danger of contamination of wounds by unclean hands or dressings.

Contamination averted by covering with gauze, and by thoroughly washing the hands before touching wound.

Use of iodine and mercurochrome.

First aid worker expected to apply only simplest form of dressing; permanent dressing to be left to the surgeon.

Use of dressing materials in cases and cabinets.

How to treat lacerated wounds, punctured wounds, bruises, poisoned wounds.

Students should be drilled in wound dressing hints and in the use of surgically clean materials found in the cases.

Instructors should not attempt to go deeply into the subject of wound infection by germs, but should emphasize the necessity of not touching the wounds and of the use of surgically clean dressings.

Drilling in the use of the bandages should accompany this lesson.

TOPIC IV

Fractures

(Manual references—pages 25 to 32)

This lesson may be preceded by or accompanied with simple instruction as to the bony structure of the human body, joints, etc.

Varieties of fractures, their causes, symptoms and dangers.

First aid is to prevent further damage; treatment is to be left for the surgeon.

First aid workers should never attempt to set a fracture.

Necessity for excessive care in removal of clothing, and handling a fractured part.

Instruction should be given in methods of applying pads and splints to fractures in the various parts of the body, and the use of the Triangular Bandage as a support.

Students should practice the making and using of improvised splints.

Students should be instructed in the handling of compound fractures.

Dislocations —First aid consists in fixing the limb in a comfortable position, and awaiting medical aid.

Sprains and strains may be treated with cold applications, bandaging and placing the limb in a comfortable position.

TOPIC V
Burns and Scalds
(Manual references—pages 33 to 35)

The instructor should emphasize the importance of prompt action in the relief of burns, and the urgency of medical attendance when the injury is extended (second and third degree).

Treatment involves the relief of pain, and the treatment of the shock.

The pupils should practice the handling of a person whose clothes are supposed to be on fire.

They should be impressed with the use of ready-to-hand measures for covering burns and relieving pain.

Burns from acids, chemicals and electricity, as well as sunburn and frost bites, should be exemplified.

TOPIC VI
Sunstroke, Fainting Fits, Unconsciousness, Suffocation, Foreign Bodies in the Passages, Sprains, Dislocations
(Manual references—pages 51 to 58)

The necessity for coolness, judgment and decision should be urged.

The sending for a physician is all important.

The difficulty of distinguishing between the various types of unconsciousness, or insensibility, should be pointed out and a hasty conclusion guarded against.

The first aid worker may always, with safety, send for medical aid, and place the patient in a comfortable and safe position.

Pupils should be cautioned against giving stimulants in these cases.

The complication and danger of foreign bodies in the passages should be pointed out and the necessity of medical aid urged.

This last class of accidents are common in the household, and the pupils may well give special attention to them.

The first aid measures in these cases can best be taught by class practice.

TOPIC VII
Artificial Respiration
(Manual references—pages 59 to 64)

Applicable in drowning, electrical accidents, suffocation by gases and vapors, hanging, smothering, etc.

The class may be drilled in methods of rescue in drowning, gases and smoke, electricity accidents, etc. All pupils should be drilled in the Schaefer method of resuscitation.

The instructor in this lesson should be guided by the variety of suffocations which the pupils are most liable to meet, with special attention to automobile and household suffocation from gas.

TOPIC VIII
Transportation of Injured
(Manual references—pages 95 to 100)

Emphasize the point that the patient should be prepared for transportation at the place of injury.

The ordinary methods of handling and transporting patients with imaginary injuries, fractures, etc., should be learned by practice.

. If convenient, the use of litters, stretchers and carriers should be exemplified and practice lessons given.

The emergency construction of stretchers from materials found in shops, industries, along railroads, in mines, etc., should be discussed.

Where hospital facilities are not available the preparation of the room where the injury is to be cared for, should be explained.

TOPIC IX
Domestic Emergencies, Including Poisons
(Manual references—pages 103 to 118)

Urge the point that drugs are to be administered only by a physician.

First aid workers should use only simple measures which

[71]

tend to relieve the patient until the arrival of medical aid.

The class should not attempt to memorize the poisons or antidotes; better rely upon the book. They should, however, become familiar with the general measures.

First aid workers should not administer antidotes when medical aid can be obtained.

Emetics are a safe procedure in cases where indicated.

Essentials of First Aid

First Aid is the rendering of immediate and efficient assistance in accidents and sudden injury.

The principal objects of first aid are:

Relief from immediate danger; prevention from further injury; placing the patient under medical care.

To render efficient first aid the worker must have knowledge, common sense, and experience. These are acquired by study and practice.

The first aid student should be observant—noting the cause and signs of injury.

Tactful—avoiding thoughtless questions and learning the symptoms and history of the case.

Resourceful—using whatever is at hand to the best advantage so as to prevent further damage.

Explicit—giving clear instructions to the patient, and advice to the assistants.

Discriminating—that he may decide which of the several injuries should be given attention.

REQUIREMENTS FOR FIRST AID AND MEDICAL
SERVICE IN INDUSTRY

THE suggestions which follow are based upon observations made during a survey conducted by the Research Staff of the publishers of this Manual, covering a large number of industries of the United States. The survey was made to ascertain the methods employed in the industries in applying first aid measures to injured employees, and also included the service rendered to employees in the treatment of injuries, following the preliminary measures of first aid.

The suggestions are of necessity given in condensed form. They may be taken in part as the opinions of the observer, supplemented by the suggestions of industrial surgeons and workers in the medical service in the industries under review.

In the main the suggestions are based upon the service in actual use in the industries under survey. Added to these are suggestions looking toward an adequate medical service in industries of various sizes and types.

The suggestions are intended to cover industrial plants from the smallest to the largest.

In these recommendations, it is to be noted that all types of industry cannot be included. For example, department stores must give stress to rest rooms rather than to surgical facilities. In many industries there is little need for X-ray and physiotherapy departments or for operating rooms. In the case of railroads, where large numbers are employed, it is difficult to formulate specific suggestions. In certain instances, the railway companies and other industries maintain their own hospitals, thus doing away with the problem of equipment. In most instances, railways maintain dispensaries at shops or terminals for emergency cases.

The hospital, dispensary and first aid room have proven to be a necessity in many industries. Their development has been due to progress and increased efficiency, coupled with a humanitarian spirit, more than the various laws that have been enacted by the states.

The success of the dispensary, hospital or first aid room depends not only on the equipment, number of rooms and large personnel, but on the relation between the employees and the dispensary attendant, whether physician, nurse or first aid worker.

The hospital, dispensary or first aid room should be an integral part of the plant in spirit as well as in part. A closer bond between this department and all of the employees should be encouraged, cultivated and established.

Equipment Under 100 Employees

A plant employing less than 100 people can satisfy the first aid and medical needs of its employees with the use of a suitable first aid cabinet. It is advisable, however, in places employing even this number to set aside a suitable room for the purpose. If an allotment of such space is impossible, then the office of the plant may be used. It is inadvisable to treat injuries in the work rooms of the factory.

In certain types of industry an excess of splints, bandages, etc., will be found advantageous. Where women employees predominate, suitable medicines may be needed. Very little equipment outside of the necessary articles need be kept—a table, two chairs, a cot, glazed sink, supply of towels and soap, and a blanket or two will usually suffice. A stretcher should be available.

100 to 300 Employees

This number would require a moderate sized room with a floor space of approximately 200 square feet, divided by a partition. This room should be centrally located, and afford the patients privacy and comfort. It should be well supplied with light, heat, and good ventilation. It is recommended that the floor be of impervious material such as linoleum, tile, magnesite, etc., and that the walls be painted, preferably a shade of green, otherwise white or light tan.

The equipment should include the following: glazed sink with hot and cold running water; sterilizer; table with smooth top; two or more chairs; a couch or a bed with two pillows; two woolen blankets; heavy rubber sheet; waste receptacle; stretcher; enameled wash basins; hot water bottle; individual drinking cups; desks for doctor and nurse. A first aid cabinet should be maintained with such additional supplies as may be found necessary. Simple medicines for common ailments, colds, etc., may be kept at hand.

300 to 500 Employees

Two rooms should be available. One room, small in size, to be used as a waiting room. The second or larger may be divided into two parts—the smaller part to be used for physical examinations, and the second part for treatments and dressings. The type of floor and color scheme are identical with the foregoing.

The dispensary proper should contain a nurse's desk; table for dressings; a chair with a head-rest for eye work; adjustable light; sterilizer; glazed sink; chairs with arm-rests; foot-rests; arm and foot basins; waste pail; stool; a cot; a closet for medicinal and surgical supplies, a cabinet for surgical instruments; blankets, pillows, splints.

500 to 1,000 Employees

Three rooms are usually required—the first a small waiting room, the second room for physical examinations, and the third for treatment and dressings. If the number of employees reaches toward 1,000, and the service is active, it will be advisable to supply an additional room which, when required, may be used as a hospital rest room for severe cases.

The equipment needed is of necessity more elaborate than that noted in the foregoing section. The waiting room should provide ample seating capacity, as well as the nurse's desk. The surgical room should be large and should carry equipment similar to those industries employing 300 to 500, but in greater amounts.

1,000 to 2,000 Employees

The layout here depends chiefly on three factors—first, the nature of the industry, second, the location of the plant, and third, the type of service which it is to maintain. Where possible, it is advisable to maintain a dispensary in a separate building, especially so in the case of hazardous industries. The minimum number of rooms should be four. It is advisable to include (1) a waiting room; (2) physician's office; (3) nurse's office, which can also be used for the keeping of records; (4) a main surgical room; (5) physical examination room; (6) small laboratory; (7) dental department. If the medical service is extended, an X-ray room, a physiotherapy room and a hospital rest room may also be maintained.

The main surgical room should be equipped as outlined in previous sections, with the addition of an adjustable operating table. An instrument cabinet should be provided, also surgical and medical supplies and equipment in quantity to supply the increased number of cases. A small laboratory may be equipped for urine analysis.

2,000 to 5,000 Employees

The layout here is similar to the one for 1,000 to 2,000 employees, except for increased space. Based upon observations made during the survey, the arrangement should be somewhat as follows: (1) waiting room; (2) doctor's office; (3) nurse's office; (4) physical examination room; (5) two surgical rooms, one for clean and one for infected cases; (6) X-ray and dark rooms; (7) physiotherapy room; (8) laboratory; (9) hospital room for severely injured cases; (10) lavatories; (11) dental office. Minor surgery may be carried on here, even if hospital facilities are at some short distance. When the plant buildings are scattered, it is at times necessary to have a dispensary in one of the outside buildings. The color schemes, types of floor and the necessary facilities for light, heat and ventilation are the same as heretofore noted.

The laboratory should be equipped to do ordinary urine

analysis and blood counts. Laboratory work can be extended to include the Wassermann test and sputum examinations.

Where a branch dispensary is maintained, this room should have simple equipment with supplies of small dressings to meet the needs. Important cases should always be treated at the main dispensary.

5,000 to 10,000 Employees

The layout here is the same as in the foregoing, except that additional rooms are necessary where the number of cases treated is large. Where the nature of the work is hazardous and the plant is not located near a hospital, the company may maintain its own hospital.

The rooms and the equipment may follow the treatment noted in the previous section.

The equipment in a large industry such as this must be extensive, especially if the number of cases treated per day runs high. Where possible, it is advisable to have an entire building devoted to the medical department.

If the plant is situated at a distance from hospital service, it may be advisable to be equipped to perform operations reaching to major surgery.

A physiotherapy room may be provided. A room may be needed for eye, ear, nose and throat work, and should be painted black. A laboratory should be maintained, equipped for routine urine analysis and blood work. If desired, the apparatus can be provided to include sputum examinations and Wassermann tests.

A room may be devoted to the keeping of records.

Over 10,000 Employees

Specific details as to layout in such an industry will vary with the nature of the industry, severity and frequency of accidents, location of plant, etc. It is advisable that an entire building be devoted to the medical department, especially where the industry is of the hazardous or "heavy" type. It should contain

(1) waiting room; (2) large surgical dressing room; (3) room for eye, ear, nose and throat service; (4) dental room; (5) operating room for major cases; (6) operating room for minor cases; (7) hospital ward for women; (8) hospital ward for men; (9) X-ray department; (10) examination booths or rooms; (11) physiotherapy department; (12) laboratory; (13) dietitian's room.

Increase in the number of employees does not materially change the principle governing the equipment of the medical service in industries. The larger the number of employees to be cared for, together with the nature of the work, will govern the equipment. The equipment noted in the preceding section will apply to many industries employing over 10,000 except that, as the number rises, greater capacity and more apparatus are needed.

Important adjuncts to any hospital department of a fair-sized plant are apparatus that have proven useful in resuscitation. Among these may be included the oxygen tank and the new type of inhalator (oxygen and carbon dioxide).

Other important articles of equipment are the apparatus necessary for blood transfusion, and for forcing fluids into the body (hypodermoclysis).

Medical Staff and Service

Usually in industries there are three different individuals who attend to injuries, viz: the physician, the nurse, first aid worker.

Regardless of the number of employees, no industry can dispense with the services of a physician.

Equitable arrangements for plants employing 300 or less are (1) The Industrial Medical Service Bureaus, (2) "Pro Rata" Dispensaries, (3) The "Single Fee Basis," and (4) Physicians "On call" only.

Industrial Medical Service Bureaus maintain a medical and surgical service, supervise the first aid activities and advise as to the equipment, etc. All injuries are sent to a dispensary maintained by the service bureau. For cases of severe injuries, the bureaus maintain their own ambulances, the patients being cared for in a hospital. The bureau assigns physicians who make periodical calls to the industries under their charge. Nurses receive instructions from the physicians of the bureau.

The "Pro Rata" Dispensary is an arrangement whereby several establishments within the same building, or plants closely related, establish a dispensary and employ physicians who will supply medical service on a "pro rata" basis.

A third method of medical service applicable to small plants is an arrangement carried out on a fee basis; under this plan a physician receives a fee from the employer for visiting the plant daily. The fourth method is the plan by which a designated physician attends only when summoned.

To summarize the requirements of industries as to medical service, it may be stated that (1) all plants should have medical service; (2) that the smaller plants may have the services of a part time physician, whether it be through the Industrial Medical Service Bureau, through a pro rata arrangement, or whether they engage a physician to make stated calls; (3) that a plant employing 1,000 or more will probably have work sufficient to require a full time physician (or two part time physicians); (4) that where the work is hazardous even 500 employees may require the services of one full time or two part time physicians, and lastly, that in general the part time physician arrangement has been more satisfactory than the full time, except in the instances enumerated, i. e., chief surgeons of railroads and large industries, chief surgeons of large plants in which administrative work is needed, and in plants remote from hospital facilities.

Nurse

It is difficult to name the minimum number of employees that may require a nurse. This depends upon the type of the industry and the frequency of the accidents. Observers have stated that all places employing over 150 should employ a full time nurse. Places employing as few as 100 might afford the services of a nurse, if the number of injuries is large. The necessity of employing a full time nurse may be governed by the number of cases of injury at a given plant.

Dental Service—Oculist Service

In the opinion of observers, industries employing 1,500 or more may well secure the services of a dentist. Smaller organizations may secure the services of a dentist who will call at intervals.

The employment of an oculist is important, especially so where eye hazards are present. Interference by a person not versed with the anatomy of the eye has led to irreparable injury, and the value of the eye is sufficiently high to place this service in the hands of an ophthalmologist who visits the plant daily, or is summoned when necessary.

Physical Examination

The question of physical examination has become prominent within the last few years. The examination of new employees is quite commonly in vogue. Periodic examination remains on debatable ground, many employers believe that periodic examinations are unnecessary. It is urged that the benefits derived from periodic examination favor the employer and the employee alike.

The intervals at which the periodic examinations should be carried on are determined by the nature of the industry and by the specific work of the employee. Employees handling food should be examined at frequent intervals, with special attention directed to venereal diseases. Men whose work depends upon their vision should have their eyes tested frequently. Men who are employed in extremely hazardous industries, should be given inspections frequently to forestall any onset of occupational disease.

First Aid by the Layman

The status of the first aid man is not clearly defined. There are instances where such a person is useful, and in many instances absolutely necessary. In a plant that is centralized and carries a suitable medical staff, the duties of the first aid man are of a minor character. The functions and duties of a first aid man as related to the treatment of injuries are: that he shall have had some training, that he acts under the supervision of the attending physician, and that he should confine his activities towards making the patient comfortable until medical aid is available.

In small establishments where a physician calls only when needed, and where the work is too small to employ a nurse, the first aid man will, of necessity, be called upon to render aid to the injured while waiting for medical aid. The training of the first aid workers is discussed elsewhere.

The thousands of employees of telephone and telegraph companies and like industries, who work far away from any medical attention, cannot be accompanied by a physician who would care for their injuries. The same is true in the mining industry.

At the National Safety Council Congress in Detroit, 1926, one physician remarked that it would be of value to have all households, all vehicles and automobiles supplied with first aid outfits, that the hazards on the highways, homes, etc., are so great that pedestrians should carry pocket kits.

It is important that the layman be in some measure qualified to attend to injuries and that he has received at least an elementary instruction in first aid. In most of the industries, courses in first aid are given to the employees.

In many lines of industry, the percentage of first aid training is increasing. It is true, however, that in certain industries, well equipped with a medical staff, first aid training of the layman has been abandoned. The fact that the employee is trained in first aid does not require him to attend to the injuries in a place where medical service is at hand.

First aid training of the layman is generally carried out in two ways. In some industries, employees are taken in groups, organized into teams, and trained. First aid contests are held, and the respective teams remain as units.

The course usually covers the treatment for the most common injuries and can be summarized as follows: (1) how to treat hemorrhage; (2) how to treat asphyxia from gas, electricity, drowning, etc.; (3) the commonest forms of splinting; (4) what not to do. The men are warned against giving anything by mouth. They are drilled in the prone pressure method of resuscitation (Schaefer Method) and it is of common report that these men are more skillful in this work (resuscitation) than many physicians.

In some industries, the layman is not permitted to treat wounds, and his activities are confined to resuscitation alone.

Rest Rooms

The rest room, in the opinion of many, is as important as the surgical dressing room. In plants that employ a large percentage of women, it is found that many ailments are relieved by an hour's stay in the quiet and comfort of the rest room.

Ordinarily, a rest room is associated with female employees, yet, there is reason to believe that rest rooms for men are an important adjunct.

Welfare

The importance of a welfare program is evident, especially in plants employing large numbers. A welfare program is unlimited, and may include:

Visiting Nurse: The duty of this nurse is to visit the home, to see the injured who is convalescing, to view conditions at the home, and to report any needs of the family of the injured employee.

Social Service: The duties are similar to those of the visiting nurse.

Publications: As a part of the welfare program, a publication, weekly, monthly or otherwise, will tend to arouse a community spirit among employees.

Educational: Certain industries maintain educational facilities.

The employee is permitted to study in his spare time and to equip himself with sufficient knowledge to be in line for advancement.

Monetary or Emolumental: These include sick benefits, pensions, etc.

Recreational: Athletic work, outings, and recreational activities of all types.

Accident Records

1. Importance of Proper Methods of Keeping and Compiling Accident Records:

(a) To maintain interest in accident prevention
(b) To show where safety work is required

2. Collecting Accident Records.

(a) Cooperation of safety, medical, operating and employment departments
(b) Suggested forms:
  (1) Daily record of all accidents
  (2) Notice of injury to employee
  (3) Foreman's report
  (4) Hospital records
  (5) Return to work notice

3. Tabulation of Accident Records.

(a) Uniform system should be followed in all industries and plants
(b) Definite tabulation of accidents
(c) Accident charts should show:
  (1) Accident frequency. (Accident frequency should be expressed in terms of the number of accidents per 1,000,000 hours worked.)
  (2) Accident Severity. (Accident severity should be expressed in terms of days lost per 1,000 hours worked, not in wages lost. The scale of time losses for death and permanent disabilities, adopted by the International Association of Industrial Accident Boards and Commissions, will be found in Bulletin No. 234, of the U. S. Bureau of Labor Statistics, page 278, or in the "Monthly Review" of the same Bureau, for October, 1917.

ELECTRIC SHOCK

R ULES recommended by the Commission on Resuscitation from Electric Shock, representing the American Medical Association, the National Electric Light Association and the American Institute of Electrical Engineers, issued by the National Electric Light Association, Engineering Societies Building, New York:

An accidental electric shock usually does not kill at once, but may only stun the victim and for a while stop his breathing.

Hope of restoring the victim lies in prompt and continued use of artificial respiration.

Instructions for Resuscitation

Follow these instructions even if the victim appears dead.

I. *Free the victim from the circuit immediately.*

1. With a single quick motion, separate the victim from the live conductor.

Observe the following precautions:

(a) Use a dry coat, a dry rope, a dry stick or board, or any other dry non-conductor to move either the victim or the wire, so as to break the electrical contact. Beware of using metal or any moist material. The victim's loose clothing, if dry, may be used to pull him away; do not touch the soles or heels of his shoes while he remains in contact—the nails are dangerous.

(b) If the body must be touched by your hands, be sure to cover them with rubber gloves, mackintosh, rubber sheeting or dry cloth; or stand on a dry board or on some other dry insulating surface. If possible, use only one hand.

If the victim is conducting the current to ground, and is convulsively clutching the live conductor, it may be easier to shut off the current by lifting him than by leaving him on the ground and trying to break his grasp.

2. Open the nearest switch, if that is the quickest way to break the circuit.

3. If necessary to cut a live wire, use an ax or a hatchet with a dry wooden handle, or properly insulated pliers.

II. *Send for the nearest doctor.*

III. *Without waiting for the doctor, start artificial respiration.*

1. As soon as the victim is clear of the live conductor, quickly feel with your finger in his mouth and throat and remove any foreign body (tobacco, false teeth, etc.). Then begin artificial respiration. Do not stop to loosen the patient's clothing; every moment of delay is serious.

Begin artificial respiration *at once.* Use the Schaefer or prone method (page 60).

If possible, avoid laying the subject so that any burned places are pressed upon.

Do not permit bystanders to crowd about and shut off fresh air.

While this is being done, an assistant should loosen any tight clothing about the subject's neck, chest, or waist.

Continue artificial respiration (if necessary, two or three hours or longer) without interruption, until natural breathing is restored.

When the doctor arrives, continue the respiration movements until the doctor stops them.

Even after natural breathing begins, carefully watch that it continues. If it stops, start artificial respiration again.

During the period of operation, keep the subject warm by applying a proper covering and by laying beside his body bottles or rubber bags filled with warm (not hot) water. The attention to keeping the subject warm should be given by an assistant or assistants.

Do not give any liquids whatever by mouth until the subject is fully conscious.

When breathing is restored the movements can be stopped. Then, and not until then, start the rubbing of the legs and arms toward the heart to restore the circulation.

After the patient becomes conscious, give him half a tea-spoonful of aromatic spirit of ammonia in a third of a glass of water. Surround him with bottles of hot water, and cover him with a blanket.

Persons shocked by electricity need fresh air.

Electric shocks are often accompanied by various types of burns, which should be treated as ordinary burns.

Burns of Eyes—At the General Electric Company works, Schenectady, N. Y., it is the practice to immediately bathe an eye affected by electric flash with witch hazel. In other establishments electrically burnt eyes are dressed with gauze dipped in sweet oil.

ACCIDENTS CAUSED BY ELECTRICITY

Accidents due to electricity are of frequent occurrence. Ordinary trolley and lighting system wires carry high voltage of the powerful current. Contact with them causes most dangerous shock and often death.

In handling electrical apparatus every operative should have before him the caution—safety first.

The avoidance of electrical accidents is fairly easy of accomplishment; the restoration of the injured patient is not easy.

"Rubber gloves should be provided by the employer and used on both hands in the handling of cables and wires, whether the parts are 'live' or not. The workman should satisfy himself before beginning work that the gloves are in good condition, Working on 'live' circuits, especially alternating current, should be avoided as far as is practicable. A man should not work on wire or conductors of any kind with sleeves rolled up or arms exposed, nor should wires ever be handled while standing or sitting in a wet place without extra precaution to obtain insulation from the ground. In handling any circuit over 115 volts known to be 'live,' it is best, if possible, to use only one hand. Keep the other in the pocket or behind the back.

"If the power has been cut off by opening a switch located some distance from where the work is being done, a sign should be always placed on the switch stating that men are working on the line.

"No examinations, repairs, or alterations, necessitating the handling of cables, wires, machines, or other apparatus under high voltage, should be made if it is possible to avoid so doing. In any case such work should be done only by a trained electrician."—Extract from a pamphlet issued by The Fidelity & Casualty Company of New York.

AMMONIA ACCIDENTS

Ammonia gas used in refrigeration plants is at times the origin of serious accidents.

Ammonia causes irritation and congestion of the lungs and bronchial organs, violent coughing and vomiting and, when breathed in sufficient quantity, suffocation. Liquid anhydrous ammonia by freezing, produces a condition which has much the same effect as severe burns caused by acid or scalding water.

In cases of partial or total suffocation by ammonia gas, remove the victim from gaseous atmosphere at once, carry to fresh moving air if possible, and immediately give artificial respiration. (Schaefer method.) Do not stop to loosen clothing, as every moment of delay is serious. Send for a doctor at once.

After starting artificial respiration, the clothing should be loosened, as well as any other restriction to the breathing.

Do not give the patient any liquid by mouth until fully conscious, after which give mild stimulants and mildly acid drinks (vinegar in water, or lemonade). Keep the body warm and give the patient plenty of fresh air at all times.

If the injury is external in the form of a freezing, or, as it is sometimes called, burning, lint, gauze or cotton dripping wet with carron oil should be applied frequently.

If the ammonia has penetrated through the clothing, the clothing should be removed at once, since it acts as a reservoir, the same as with scalding hot water or steam.

For the Eyes—First, pour a one per cent solution of boracic acid into the eyes, instructing patient to open and close the lids repeatedly, to bring the liquid in contact with the entire inner surface.

Second, after thoroughly washing the eyes, place a small quantity of clean, plain vaseline under the lids, by pulling down the lower lid and applying the vaseline with a small match-shaped piece of wood, having smooth rounded ends.

For Nose and Throat—Dip a handkerchief, or a piece of

gauze folded once, in vinegar. Wring out lightly and lay over nose and mouth. If liquid ammonia has entered the nose, snuff up some vinegar and apply sweet oil with a feather or cotton to inner surface of nostrils.

If ammonia has been swallowed, administer diluted vinegar, orange or lemon juice in liberal quantities, following up with one to four teaspoonfuls of sweet oil, milk or the whites of three or four eggs with cracked ice. If vomiting is present, aid it by liberal draughts of lukewarm water.

First Aid Don'ts

Don't touch a wound with your fingers or any instrument.
Don't put an unclean dressing or cloth over a wound.
Don't allow bleeding to go unchecked.
Don't move a patient unnecessarily.
Don't allow a patient with a fracture or suspected fracture to be moved until splints have been applied.
Don't neglect shock.
Don't burn a patient with an unwrapped hot-water bottle or other heated object.
Don't fail to give artificial respiration when needed.
Don't fail to remove false teeth, tobacco, and chewing gum from the mouth of an unconscious person.
Don't permit air to reach a burned surface.
Don't wash wounds.
Don't reduce dislocations, except of the finger and lower jaw.
Don't put a quid of tobacco on a wound.
Don't leave a tourniquet on over 20 minutes without loosening.
Don't forget to send for a physician.

GAS ASPHYXIATION

POISONING from the effects of illuminating or heating gas is frequent among workers for gas companies, public service corporations, and of occasional occurrence in ordinary households from gas stoves and heaters, defective burners, etc.

Gas from coal heating furnaces and stoves, illuminating gas and gas used for heating, smoke from fires, exhaust gases from automobiles are poisonous when breathed into the body. They contain a substance known as carbon monoxide which combines with the blood. A small amount of this poison when taken into the blood will kill. If the patient does not die in the gas, but is removed to fresh air, he may recover.

In gas poisoning first aid measures must be prompt and correct.

The methods here given are based upon the Rules for First Aid and Resuscitation in Gas Asphyxiation, recommended by the Commission on Resuscitation from Gas Asphyxiation, representing the American Gas Association.

Commission on Resuscitation from Gas Asphyxiation

DR. WALTER B. CANNON
Professor of Physiology, Medical School of Harvard University

DR. DAVID L. EDSALL
Dean, Medical School of Harvard University and Professor of Clinical Medicine, Medical School of Harvard University

DR. HOWARD W. HAGGARD
Instructor in Applied Physiology, Yale University, Consulting Physiologist to the United States Bureau of Mines

DR. LAWRENCE J. HENDERSON
Professor of Biological Chemistry, Medical School of Harvard University

DR. YANDELL HENDERSON
Professor of Applied Physiology, Yale University, Consulting Physiologist to the United States Bureau of Mines

DR. FRANCIS W. PEABODY
Professor of Medicine, Medical School of Harvard University

DR. ROYD R. SAYERS
Chief Surgeon, United States Bureau of Mines, Surgeon, United States Public Health Service

MR. CHARLES B. SCOTT
Accident Prevention Committee, American Gas Association

DR. CECIL K. DRINKER
Chairman; Associate Professor of Applied Physiology, Medical School of Harvard University

When a person is overcome by gas, the first thing to do is to get him into fresh air quickly. This may not necessarily be outdoor air, but a room or place free from gas, and in cold weather it should be a place comfortably warm.

If the rescuer has to go into the gas to get a victim, he should protect himself as far as possible, open doors and smash windows to let in fresh air, get in and get out quickly. Handkerchiefs and ordinary masks are of no use—many of them are dangerous in gas accidents, as they do not stop the carbon monoxide poison. Lives of rescuers have been lost by a feeling of false security when using an improper mask.

Gas companies usually have at hand masks and breathing apparatus specially made and filled with chemicals to combat gas poisons. These, or an oxygen breathing apparatus, are the only apparatus which are safe and sure.

Do not wait for masks, apparatus, or even for assistance, get the victim out of the gas.

If the patient is breathing, he should be placed on his stomach as shown in Fig. 88 (the first position for applying artificial respiration).

Send for a doctor and other help.

Watch the patient carefully. Do not allow him to make any exertion. Keep him lying down. If he must be moved, carry him, do not let him walk.

If inhalant apparatus for applying oxygen-carbon-dioxide can be secured, it may be used. Inhalant treatment may be started as soon as the patient is removed from the gas. The inhalant treatment is to be given at the same time artificial respiration is being carried out. Public Service and Gas Companies and sometimes Fire Departments have at hand inhalant apparatus available for use.

Pulmotors and similar mechanical apparatus for artificial respiration have been discredited and should not be used.

If the patient is not breathing, artificial respiration should be started at once.

As soon as the patient is clear of the gas quickly feel with your finger in his mouth and throat and remove any foreign body (tobacco, false teeth, etc.). If the mouth is tight shut, pay no more attention to it until later. Do not stop to loosen the patient's clothing, but immediately begin actual resuscitation. Every moment of delay is serious. Proceed as follows:

Lay the patient on his stomach, one arm extended directly overhead, the other bent at elbow and with face to one side, resting on the hand or forearm, so that the nose and mouth are free for breathing.

Start artificial respiration by the prone pressure method, proceeding as outlined on Pages 60-64 of this Manual.

Do not stop or interrupt resuscitation until stiffening of the body (rigor mortis) sets in. Lives have been saved after four hours or longer. If necessary to change operators during the attempts at resuscitation, each operator should retain the same stroke or rhythm.

If natural breathing stops after being restored, start resuscitation again.

Continue resuscitation until the patient is conscious and breathing well.

Care of the Patient

A chill may kill him or help to cause pneumonia. Wrap him in blankets and use hot water bottles or hot bricks. You can fill a hot water bottle from the radiator of an automobile. Be careful to protect the patient from burns by hot water bottles or bricks against the bare skin. An unconscious man has no way of telling you when he is being burned. A burn may be worse than the after effects of the gas. Never give an unconscious man anything to drink. It may choke him. Never give whisky. It makes a gassed man worse. Hot black coffee is excellent if the man is conscious enough to drink it. When the patient has become conscious keep him wrapped up warmly.

After the patient is conscious, give him half a teaspoonful of aromatic spirit of ammonia in a third of a glass of water. Then cover him with a coat and watch him, as a relapse may follow.

The patient must be kept quiet. He may want to get up or struggle. Keep him down. After he is conscious and breathing he may be turned on his back, if it would make him more comfortable. He must be kept lying down for at least six hours, if he tries to walk he may collapse. If possible, transport to home or hospital on a stretcher or in an ambulance.

AUTOMOBILE GAS POISONING

Of recent years, owing to the remarkable increase in the use of the automobile, and the custom of keeping them in small private garages, generally unheated, there are continually occurring cases of carbon monoxide poisoning due to allowing the motor to run in the closed garage.

This gas is odorless and tasteless and its effects are insidious and rapid. A person is overcome so suddenly that he is unable to crawl away.

The symptoms are: unconsciousness and semi-unconsciousness, patient very weak and breathing rapid but weak.

The treatment for this poisoning is to get the patient into fresh moving air as quickly as possible, send for a doctor and commence at once restorative activities, using the Schaefer method of resuscitation and the same procedure as with illuminating gas.

DROWNING ACCIDENTS

INASMUCH as many lives are lost by drowning, it is suggested that all persons living in localities where such accidents are liable to occur, acquaint themselves with simple and effectual methods of rescue and restoration. A practical way to do this is for two or more persons to go through the movements, one acting as patient, the others as rescuers.

In such organizations as the Boy and Girl Scouts, Y. M. C. A., etc., the rescue of drowning persons and methods of restoration of breathing should be taught.

Do not touch the drowning person while violently struggling in the water, but take the first opportunity to seize him, by the hair if possible, and throw him quickly on his back. Swim on your back, towing the body after you. Hold the head with one arm, so that the other arm and legs may be free. This position may be maintained longer, and the body supported more easily, until further aid from shore is received, than by breasting the waters in the usual position.

When the current sets from the land, as in sea bathing, it is better to adopt the position last described, and await aid, than to struggle for shore against the current, for this latter procedure often costs the life of both the rescuer and the one he sought to save, through ineffectual efforts that result in exhaustion.

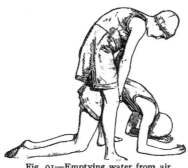

Fig. 91—Emptying water from air passages.

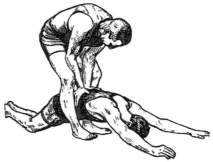

Fig. 92—Method of emptying water from air passages. Raise the body, pressing on small of back for half a minute to start ejection of water.

If a boat is available, the proper place to get bodies into the boat with the least danger of capsizing is the stern, if a dory, take in over the sides, never over the bow. The patient, in the boat or ashore, should be placed with the head lower than the chest. This may be done by laying the patient on his stomach.

This usually results in emptying, by the mouth and nostrils, much of the water that is interfering with respiration.

Restoration of Breathing

Loosen the clothing about the neck and chest, exposing them to the wind, except in very severe weather. Get the water out of the body as shown in Figs. 91 and 92.

Send for a doctor and begin artificial respiration using the Schaefer method.

Rules in Drowning Accidents

Do not let him cling around your neck or arms to endanger you.

Duck him under the water, if necessary until he is unconscious, to loosen a dangerous hold upon you. Do not strike.

Loosen clothing. Clear mouth and secure hold on tongue.

Clear air passages. Start artificial respiration. Don't hurry breathing movements; take four or five seconds for each.

Apply warmth and friction; when the patient is conscious, give hot water, coffee or hot lemonade.

Artificial breathing is of first importance. Don't give up. Persons have been revived after three or four hours of steady work.

How to Keep from Drowning

To keep from drowning it is not necessary to know how to swim. In nine cases out of ten, the knowledge of how to sustain the weight is all that is necessary to keep one's head above water.

One finger placed upon a stool, chair, small box or piece of board will easily keep the head above water, while the feet or other hand may be used as paddles to propel towards the shore.

TRANSPORTATION OF THE INJURED

Accidents often occur in places where it becomes necessary to carry the injured person to his home or to a hospital. Great care should be taken that the patient does not receive any further injury during the transportation.

Before attempting to move the patient all necessary first aid measures should be applied, and the patient carefully prepared for being moved.

Serious cases should be carried on a stretcher, which in emergency may be improvised. In absence of a stretcher various methods of transportation have been devised, some of which are here given.

The four-handed seat is made by two persons clasping each other's wrists, as shown in Fig. 93. Each person's left hand grasps his own right wrist, and the right hand of each grasps the other's left wrist.

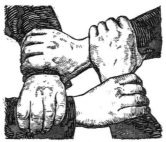

Fig. 93—Four-handed seat.

After the hands are clasped together, the bearers stoop down behind the patient, who sits on their hands, and at the same time he places one arm around the neck of each bearer.

The plan of carrying the patient by the arms and legs with the face downward, commonly called "frog's march," must never be used, as death may ensue from this treatment.

When a proper stretcher cannot be obtained, a temporary one may be made. Turn the sleeves of two coats inside out and

{95}

button the coats over them. Pass two stout poles through the sleeves. The backs of the coats form the top of the litter.

Take two sacks, make a hole in each corner of the bottoms, and pass two poles through the sacks and out of the holes.

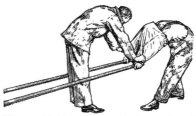

Fig. 94—Making an improvised stretcher of coats and poles.

A broad board or shutter may be employed as a stretcher; but if either of them be used, some straw, hay, blankets, or clothing should be placed on it, and covered with a piece of stout cloth, a blanket, or sacking. The sacking is useful in taking the patient off the stretcher when he arrives at the bedside.

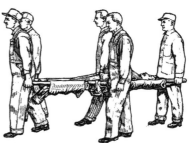

Fig. 95—An improvised "coat stretcher." Three coats have been used.

Always test a stretcher before placing the patient on it. Place an uninjured bystander upon it and spring him up and down.

To place the patient on a stretcher, put the stretcher at his head in line with the body. Let the two bearers, on opposite sides of the patient, grasp hands beneath his back and hips, raise him, lift him backwards over the stretcher and lower him upon it.

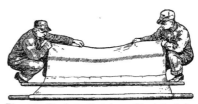

Fig. 96—Blanket stretcher. Blanket being folded on poles.

Bearers of stretchers must not keep step in marching. Opposite feet must be put forward at the same time to prevent the swaying of the stretcher and

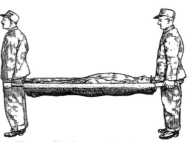

Fig. 97—Blanket stretcher. Completed.

the rolling of the patient. Never allow a stretcher to be carried on the bearers' shoulders.

Always carry the patient feet foremost, except when going up a hill. In cases of fractured thigh or fractured leg, if the patient has to be carried downhill, carry him head first.

In carrying a patient on a stretcher, avoid lifting the stretcher over walls, hedges, or ditches.

To transport the patient the bearers kneel, the right bearer on his left knee, the left bearer on his right knee; the cylinder is pulled apart so as to form a sitting space of six or eight inches between the rolls, and the patient, supported by the arms of the bearers, is placed upon this space for transportation. By this method one arm of each bearer is free for any emergency.

The methods of transportation illustrated in this section need no explanation. They were specially posed under the direction of experienced first aid instructors and trainers.

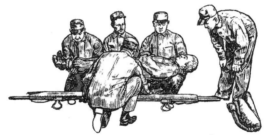

Fig. 98—Placing injured patient on a stretcher.

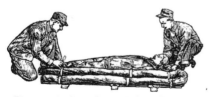

Fig. 99—Broken Back Splint. Padded splints placed under patient.

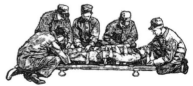

Fig. 100—Broken Back Splint. Patient tied to the splint and then placed on a stretcher. Note that the hands are held in a loose sling.

ONE MAN CARRY ON BACK

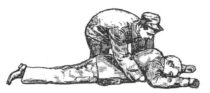

Fig. 101—First method of lifting.

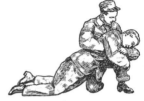

Fig. 102—Second method of lifting.

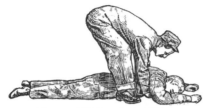

Fig. 103—Third method of lifting.

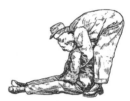

Fig. 104—Fourth method of lifting.

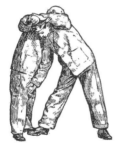

Fig. 105—The rescuer ready to lift patient from standing position to his back.

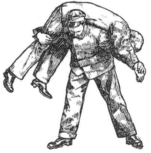

Fig. 106—Patient on back of rescuer.

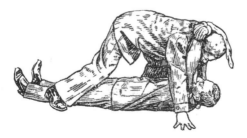

Fig. 107—Low Drag. May be used in low seam mines or buildings where the air is filled with smoke and gases. The patient's wrists are tied together with a bandage or handkerchief, and rescuer crawls toward the fresh air or exit, dragging the patient.

ONE MAN CARRY IN ARMS

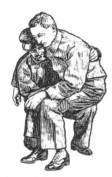
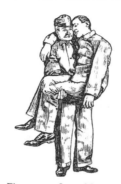
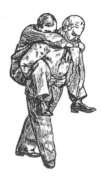

Fig. 108—One Man Carry In Arms. Second position.

Fig. 109—One Man Carry In Arms. Third position.

Fig. 110—The Morgan Carry. May be used when rescuer reaches place where he can stand erect.

THREE MEN CARRY

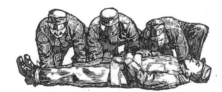

Fig. 111—Preparing to lift patient.

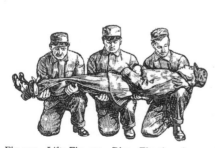
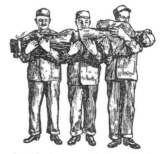

Fig. 112—Lift; Fig. 113—Rise—The three bearers kneel on the knee nearest the patient's feet and slide their hands and forearms under the patient. At the command of "Lift," they lift the patient to their knees. At the command of "Prepare to Rise," the bearers turn the patient so that he is held close to their chests and facing them. At the command "Rise," they rise to their feet.

EMERGENCY METHODS OF TRANSPORTATION

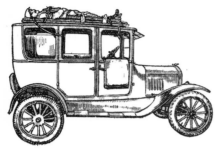

Fig. 114—Ford Sedan used as an emergency ambulance. Patient fastened to a board. The board is strapped to the top of the car. In practice the patient should be covered with a blanket.

Fig. 115—Ford Touring Car used as an emergency ambulance. Patient strapped to board and laid over the seats. In practice patient should be covered with a blanket.

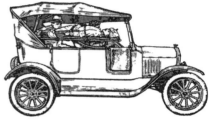

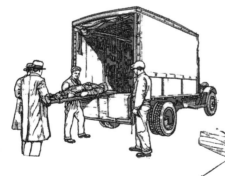

Fig. 116—Mack Truck used as an emergency ambulance. Patient strapped to improvised stretcher

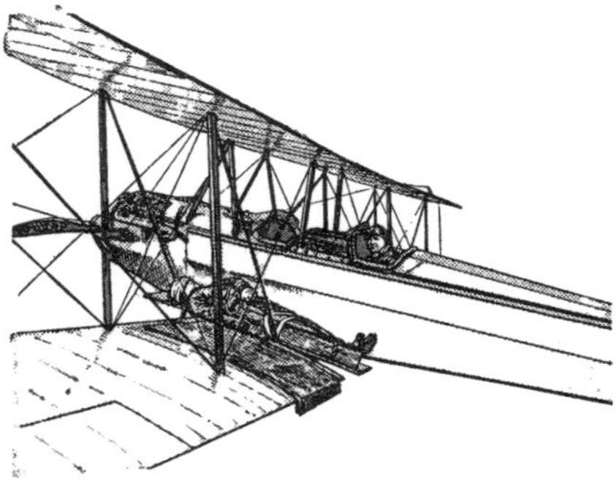

Fig. 117—Pitcairn Three Place Biplane converted into an emergency ambulance. Patient laid on a board. The board strapped to the wing. In practice the patient should be covered with a blanket.

PREPARATION FOR THE RECEPTION
OF THE INJURED

WHEN an injured or sick person is to be removed to a private house instead of to a hospital, preparations should be made, if possible, before the patient is brought in. In such preparation the following hints will be of value.

A room should be chosen which can be easily reached. The way to the room must be cleared of furniture and loose mats. If the injured person is carried on a stretcher, a couple of strong chairs should be placed ready to support it wherever the bearers might require rest. Unnecessary furniture and hangings should be removed from the room. The bed should be drawn out from the wall so that both sides can be approached, and the bed clothes turned back on one side to their full length. Several hot water bottles and hot blankets may be required.

If the injury is very severe, or if extensive dressings have to be applied, a firm, long table, covered with old sheets or waterproof material, on which to lay the patient, should be placed near the bed.

A firm mattress should be on the bed. If there is much injury, or if dressings have to be applied, a draw-sheet should be placed on the bed, over a piece of waterproof sheeting or oilcloth or newspapers.

In fracture of the leg or thigh, sprained ankle, and like cases, a "cradle" may be needed. The use of a "cradle" is to support the bedclothes and to keep them from pressing on the limb. Bandboxes, three-legged stools, and similar articles may be used. A half barrel hoop passed under the bedclothes and tied by loop made with a needle and cord will relieve the pressure of the bedclothes.

In removing clothes from an injured person it is much better to sacrifice the clothes than to run any risk of increasing the injury. In case of a fractured arm, the uninjured arm should be drawn out first. In putting garments on, the injured arm should be put in first. To remove the trousers from a severely injured limb, rip the outside seam.

A fire in the room will generally be of service, even in summer. There should be plenty of water, both hot and cold, also several basins (stoneware or enameled preferred), an abundance of clean towels and soap, slop jars or pails. The basins should be placed on a table, which should be covered with a towel. Towels folded up should be placed on the same table; hot and cold water should be within easy reach.

A new nail brush, scissors, safety pins and needles are essential.

In the case of a burn, soft cloths, old linen, oil and bicarbonate of soda (baking soda), should be ready.

In case of bleeding, gauze sponges, plenty of hot water and several basins should be at hand.

If time will allow, the room should be thoroughly cleaned, by scrubbing and dusting woodwork and walls; then well aired.

In placing a bed or cot the head should be toward a partition (inside wall), and the foot, if possible, should be toward the fire or radiator.

The bed should be high and so placed that both sides can be reached easily, and to allow a free circulation of air without a draught.

POISONS

Poisons are defined as substances which, when taken into the system in quantities larger than the ordinary dose, will produce serious disorder or death.

The signs and symptoms of poison vary with the nature of the substance and the part of the body acted upon. It is useless to attempt to remember the symptoms or the antidotes for the various poisons. There are, however, certain broad rules which the first aid worker may follow:

Always send for a physician. Tell him the name of the poison, if known.

Cause the patient to vomit, *except when the lips, tongue and throat are burned by strong acid or caustic alkali.*

To produce vomiting, tickle the throat with the forefinger; repeat this two or three times. If this measure is not successful add to a tumblerful of lukewarm water a tablespoon of salt, or a dessertspoonful of mustard, and give it to the patient to drink.

Often it is required to use all methods, and to repeat them, in order to produce vomiting.

Emetics may be procured at the drug store. Common emetics are the wine or the syrup of ipecac. Of these preparations a teaspoonful may be given to a child and a tablespoonful to an adult.

Use milk, raw eggs beaten up in water or milk, olive, salad or sweet oil (except in phosphorus poisoning), strong tea or coffee. After vomiting give demulcent drinks.

Save all vomit and excreta. Also preserve all bottles, powders, and drugs to show to the physician.

Foods often become poisoned because they develop within them certain ferments which act as poisons. The usual symptoms are pain in the stomach, vomiting, weakness, cramps, dilation of the pupils and drowsiness, which may go on to collapse. In such cases give emetics, castor oil, hot tea or coffee to drink, and apply warmth externally.

Alcohol Poisoning

The restrictions governing the sale of alcoholic beverages together with increased use of alcohol for industrial purposes has caused an increased number of cases of alcoholic poisoning.

Ethyl alcohol, also known as grain, molasses, or straight alcohol, is a poison in large doses. The first symptoms of alcoholic poisoning are a stimulation "hilarity" passing rapidly to stupor, loss of sensation and motion, and paralysis. Speech is thick, gait is uncertain, drowsiness sets in, the face changes from flushing to paleness, breathing is slow, the skin cold and blue, the pupils of the eyes are usually dilated.

Alcoholic poisoning and apoplexy at times resemble each other. Alcoholic poisoning can usually be distinguished by the odor of the breath.

The large use of wood alcohol and denatured alcohol in the arts, in rubbing alcohol, varnishes and numerous compounds for toilet and other purposes have greatly increased the number of cases of alcoholic poisoning.

Users of alcohol for any purpose should remember that wood alcohol is a deadly poison. The vapor of wood alcohol has been known to produce blindness, as well as dangerous maladies of the nerves and brain.

, The so-called "denatured" alcohols often contain virulent poisons; they should not be taken into the stomach and should always be used with caution.

Treatment of Alcoholic Poisoning—Victims of alcohol poisoning should receive prompt treatment. They should not be sent to jail as a case of drunkenness as delay might be dangerous.

Send for a doctor at once.

If the poisoning is from the vapors of alcohol, such as in the use of paints, varnishes, etc., get the patient into fresh air. If the alcohol has been swallowed, give an emetic. Keep the body warm by blankets, hot water bottles, etc. If the patient can walk, keep him moving, give him strong coffee or tea. If the victim collapses and breathing stops apply artificial respiration.

General Rules in Case of Poisoning

1. Send for a doctor at once, stating what has occurred, and if possible the name of the poison.

2. EXCEPT when the lips and mouth are stained or burned by an acid or alkali, promptly give an EMETIC—that is, make the patient vomit, by giving either:

(*a*) Mustard—a tablespoonful in a tumblerful (½ pint) of lukewarm water, and repeated until vomiting occurs, or

(*b*) Salt—two tablespoonfuls in a tumblerful (½ pint) of lukewarm water, and repeated until vomiting occurs.

If vomiting is retarded, putting the two fingers to the back of the throat may sometimes hasten it.

Poisoning by whisky, brandy, gin, or other intoxicating liquors are to be treated by the methods given elsewhere.

3. If the lips and mouth are stained or burned give NO emetic, but—

(*a*) If an Acid is known to be the poison, at once give an Alkali, such as lime-water, or a tablespoonful of whitening, chalk, magnesia, or wall plaster in a tumblerful (½ pint) of water.

(*b*) If an Alkali is known to be the poison, at once give an Acid, such as vinegar or lemon juice diluted with an equal quantity of water.

4. In all cases when the patient is not insensible give milk, raw eggs beaten up with milk or water, cream and flour beaten up together, animal or vegetable oil (except in phosphorus poisoning) and tea.

Oil is soothing, and is therefore especially useful in poisoning by acids, alkalies and such substances as arsenic and corrosive sublimate. Demulcent drinks, such as barley water or thin gruel, act in the same manner and are free from danger. In cases of phosphorus poisoning do not give oil.

These may be given either before or after the emetic if the poison calls for one.

Strong tea acts as a neutraliser of many poisons, and is always safe.

5. When a person has swallowed poison and threatens to go to sleep, keep him awake by walking him about and slapping his face, neck and chest with a wet towel. Strong black coffee may be given to drink. Slapping the soles of the feet may also be tried.

6. If the throat is so swollen as to threaten obstruction to the air passage, apply hot flannels or poultices to the front of the neck, and give frequent sips of cold drinks.

7. Apply artificial respiration if breathing cannot be discerned or is failing.

8. Treat shock and collapse.

9. Preserve any vomited matter, food or other substance suspected of being the poison. Do not wash vessels which may have contained the poison, but carefully guard them. Show them to the doctor, they may aid in determining the nature of the poison.

Certain poisons require special treatment, and a few of the commoner of these are mentioned below with their treatment.

POISONS AND ANTIDOTES

Sulphuric Acid, Muriatic Acid, Oxalic Acid, Nitric Acid

No emetic. Give one or two tablespoonsful of magnesia, chalk, soap suds, raw eggs, milk, sweet oil.

Carbolic Acid, Creosote

If detected immediately give castor oil, sweet oil, raw eggs or milk, followed by an emetic—tablespoonful of Epsom salts or Glauber salts in small tumblerful of milk or water; also mucilaginous drinks. Full strength alcohol applied promptly to external burns from carbolic acid will act as an antidote.

Prussic Acid
Cyanide of Potassium

Give stimulants freely. Give hot and cold douches; emetics.

Chloral

Give an emetic. Keep patient aroused. Apply mustard plaster over heart and calves of legs. Use artificial respiration.

Strychnine

Give strong tea and animal charcoal, and follow this by an emetic. Use artificial respiration when necessary.

Opium

Give emetics such as mustard or ipecac. Give coffee by rectum or mouth. Do not give alcoholic stimulants. Keep the patient aroused by walking, whipping or other means.

Caustic Soda, Caustic Potash

Give vinegar, juice of orange or lemon, citric or tartaric acids. Give also raw eggs, sweet oil, barley water or arrowroot gruel.

Arsenic, Paris Green

Give emetics of hot greasy water, or salt and water promptly; a large amount of magnesia, or lime scraped from the walls or ceiling. Give castor oil, sweet oil, or equal parts of sweet oil and lime water, or lime water alone, raw eggs, milk and stimulants (well diluted).

Blue Vitriol, Blue Stone

Give copious draughts of warm water and emetics; give white of eggs, milk, oils, flaxseed tea and demulcent drinks.

Corrosive Sublimate, Bichloride of Mercury

If detected immediately after swallowing, give an emetic, white of eggs, milk, mucilage, arrowroot gruel, barley water, or flour and water—and give all that the patient will swallow.

Iodine

Give any kind of starch or starch food freely; wheat, flour or arrowroot boiled in water—freely; chalk, magnesia and stimulants. Give emetics and apply external heat.

Lead—Red Lead, Sugar of Lead, White Lead, Paints

Induce vomiting. Give large doses of Epsom or Glauber salts. Apply mustard plasters to extremities. Give stimulating, sweet or mucilaginous drinks.

Phosphorus

Give emetics, followed by magnesia, white of eggs, purgatives. No fats or oils. Dash cold water on the head and spine.

Tartar Emetic

Give warm water freely. Give stimulants—strong tea or coffee, and apply warmth. Give white of eggs and soothing drinks, such as flaxseed or slippery elm tea.

Zinc—Sulphate or Chloride

Give bicarbonate of soda (baking powder in water); milk, white of eggs, mucilaginous drinks and emetics, hot tea or coffee.

Belladonna

Give emetics and stimulants. Apply warmth to extremities and mustard plasters to the feet. If the patient is insensible, use artificial respiration.

Foxglove Digitalis

Give emetics, followed by repeated draughts of strong tea. Apply mustard plaster over the heart and calves of the legs. Give stimulants internally.

Poisonous Food

Give emetics, castor oil, use coffee as a stimulant and apply heat. This treatment is applicable to poisoning by eating mussels or poisoned meat or fish, mushrooms, etc.

DOMESTIC EMERGENCIES

THIS Manual is primarily designed to meet accidents which occur in the factory and workshop or home, and does not, except incidentally, touch upon such emergencies as attacks of sudden illness. There is, however, a legitimate demand for suggestions for use in emergencies which may arise at night, when traveling, camping out or in situations where a physician cannot be summoned. The editors hold firmly to the opinion that drugs should be administered only under the direction of a physician. The suggestions which follow are therefore confined to simple measures which do not require the use of drugs. In all emergencies the first thing to do is to send for a physician.

Angina Pectoris (Painful heart attack) —Apply cold over the region of the heart. This is more grateful to some people than heat, and should be tried first. Hot applications, such as hot water bags, hot cloths and mustard plasters, may be used where cold applications fail.

Asthma—Persons susceptible to attacks of asthma should keep a supply of suitable burning or inhaling material for immediate use (asthma cigarettes). If such are not at hand, saturate a piece of blotting paper with a strong solution of saltpeter, dry and ignite it; let the patient inhale the fumes. If no other means are at hand, let the person attacked engage in some diversion that will occupy attention, such as smoking a cigar or pipe, reading a book or paper, or writing.

Colic—Apply heat in the form of hot water bags or bottles, hot plates, or mustard plaster over the seat of pain. Hot baths are sometimes beneficial. Never give a purgative except on the advice of a physician.

Cramps—Apply mustard plaster to the part affected, and to the extremities. If in muscles of leg or other muscles of the body, bathe the part in water as hot as can be borne. Cramps of the stomach are sometimes dangerous. Apply hot cloths over the stomach or mustard plasters at the pit of the stomach and the extremities.

Croup—In sudden attacks divert the patient's attention and allay his fears. Let him inhale steam from a pan of boiling water, to which lime water or a small quantity of Compound Tincture of Benzoin (Turlington's Balsam) has been added. Flannels wrung out in hot water may be applied to the throat and covered with some waterproof material. In children ½–1 teaspoonful of the syrup or wine of ipecac, to cause vomiting, may bring relief.

Membraneous croup is often diphtheria, and should be treated immediately with diphtheria antitoxin by a physician. In such cases hospitalization is recommended. As it is very difficult to distinguish beween ordinary croup and membraneous croup, summon a physician at once in every case of croup.

Diarrhea-Dysentery—Stop all foods. A mustard plaster, hot water bag, or turpentine stupe over the abdomen will tend to relieve pain. Hot drinks, such as ginger tea, peppermint, or chamomile tea may be given. After a preliminary starvation period of 12–24 hours, during which time the above hot drinks are given, hot gruel cereals may be fed. Purgatives should be administered only on the advice of a physician.

Earache—Consult a physician immediately. Warm sweet oil dropped in the ear, or an irrigation of the ear with warm boric acid solution from a sterilized fountain syringe, may give relief. A hot water bag applied over the ear may also help to alleviate the pain. The nose must likewise be treated to relieve the congestion which is always present in earache. This can be done best by a physician. Enlarged adenoids and tonsils are a frequent cause of earache.

Fever—Fever is not a disease. It is merely a symptom of a disease. When it is present absolute rest in bed is essential. Do not have the patient too warmly covered. Cooling drinks, such as orange juice, weak tea, and plenty of water may be given. An ice bag to the head may make the patient more comfortable. If the fever is extremely high, an alcohol rub or a sponge bath with water of about 90° F may be given.

Nervousness—In severe attacks, put the patient to bed; give hot drinks, such as milk or hot lemonade, but never give coffee. Apply heat or mustard to the soles of the feet, back and chest.

Hernia-Strangulated—Place the patient on his back in bed; elevate the foot of the bed about twelve inches; bend the patient's legs back toward the abdomen. Apply to the hernia towels or cloths wrung out in hot water; if these do not bring relief, use cold water. Call in a physician promptly in any case.

Hiccough—In severe attacks apply mustard plasters over the stomach. Hot vinegar, brandy or whisky applied in the same manner will sometimes bring relief. Let the patient draw a deep breath and hold it as long as possible. Let the patient take a drink of water.

Hysteria—Leave the patient alone in a well ventilated, darkened room, after seeing that he or she is comfortable and well covered.

Neuralgia—Apply a mustard plaster or hot cloths over the seat of pain. If hot applications fail to relieve, apply cold.

Retention of Urine—Apply hot cloths over bladder; give a warm sitz-bath. In some instances walking over a cold wet floor or dashing cold water on the legs and thighs, will cause a discharge and bring relief.

Vomiting—Give large amounts of hot water, as hot as can be taken; patient should always lie down. Small bits of ice held in the mouth or swallowed, will relieve vomiting caused by indigestion. A lump of ice held against the pit of the stomach will sometimes bring relief. If other means fail, apply a mustard plaster to the pit of the stomach.

SPECIAL MEASURES WITH CHILDREN

(1) If a child is suddenly attacked with vomiting, purging, and prostration, send for a doctor at once. In the meantime, put the child in a hot bath for a few minutes, then carefully dry with a warm towel, and wrap in warm blankets. If his hands and feet are cold, bottles filled with hot water and wrapped in flannel should be laid against them.

(2) A mush-poultice, or one made of flaxseed meal, to which one-quarter part of mustard flour has been added, or flannels wrung out in hot vinegar and water, should be placed over the belly.

(3) Five drops of brandy in a teaspoonful of water may be given every ten or fifteen minutes. No food should be given for 6–24 hours, except weak tea sweetened with a little sugar. Milk had best be withheld for 24 hours.

(4) If the diarrhea has just begun, or if it is caused by improper food, a teaspoonful of castor oil, or of the spiced syrup of rhubarb, should be given.

(5) If the child has been fed partly from the breast and partly on other food, the mother's milk alone may be used after a starvation period of 6–24 hours. If the child has been weaned, it may have, after the starvation period, diluted boiled milk and well-cooked cereal gruels. It may also have weak beef tea or chicken broth.

(6) The child should be allowed to drink cool boiled water freely.

(7) The soiled diapers or the discharges should at once be removed from the room, but saved for the physician to examine at his visit.

MISCELLANEOUS SUGGESTIONS

Temperature of the Sick Room—Sixty-eight to seventy degrees Fahrenheit is considered a good average temperature for the sick room. It should rarely be higher. In some respiratory diseases it is advisable to have it even lower.

When a patient is being washed or dressed, or a change is made of clothing or sheets, the temperature should be kept at seventy or thereabout. During the night and toward morning the sick or injured person is very susceptible to a change of temperature, and at that time care should be taken of the room and of the covering of the patient.

Baths—Cold baths are used to reduce fever in heat stroke and other cases where the temperature is high. The usual method is to put the patient into a bath of between seventy and eighty degrees Fahrenheit, and to reduce the temperature by adding cool water until it reaches sixty or sixty-five degrees.

, Tepid baths are those in which the temperature of the water varies from eighty to ninety degrees. In warm baths, the temperature varies from ninety to a little less than one hundred. These baths are used where there is excitement, irritability, or some affection of the nervous system.

Hot baths are useful in cases of shock, depression and similar ills. The temperature of the water in a hot bath varies from ninety-eight to one hundred and ten degrees Fahrenheit.

Upon leaving the bath the skin should be quickly dried and the patient put to bed as quickly as possible. Hot baths may produce fainting, and should always be taken in the presence of an attendant. Always use a thermometer to take the temperature of the water; the hand is very deceptive.

TEMPERATURE OF THE BODY

In health the normal temperature of the body is 98.4 degrees Fahrenheit. When the temperature is higher than this the patient is commonly said to have fever. The temperature ordinarily rises in the afternoon, being nearly a degree higher then and in the first part of the night than in the early morning. It again gradually falls from midnight to six or seven o'clock in the morning. Should the temperature of a patient taken at ten o'clock at night be one degree higher than when taken at five o'clock in the afternoon, it need not be considered an increase of fever. The temperature of children frequently rises as much as two degrees from slight causes and this in itself need occasion no alarm.

In severe shock, exposure to cold, alcoholic poisoning, etc., the temperature falls. Should the temperature in such cases fall to 96 degrees Fahrenheit or below, a physician should be summoned at once. Heat should be supplied to the body (see Shock, page 10) and hot tea or coffee given to the patient, at the same time raising the temperature of the room to above 70 degrees Fahrenheit.

To Take the Temperature—The instrument used for recording the temperature of the body is termed a clinical thermometer. The best form is self-registering, and has a lens front to magnify the mercury column. The degrees are indelibly marked on the stem, an arrow marking the degree of normal temperature.

First shake the thermometer until the mercury is below the arrow. Then, placing the bulb well back in the mouth beneath the tongue, have the patient close the lips and allow the thermometer to remain in place from two to five minutes. When it is inconvenient to take the temperature by mouth, the thermometer may be placed in the armpit, there to remain for five or six minutes. The temperature of an infant may best be taken by oiling and inserting the bulb end of the thermometer about an inch into the rectum. The rectal temperature is normally one degree higher than the mouth temperature; in an armpit, one degree lower.

The Pulse—The average pulse rate in an adult is seventy-six beats per minute. This rate varies according to age, as shown in the following table:

At birth	130–140
1st year	115–130
2d year	100–115
3d year	95–105
7–14 "	80– 90
14–21 "	75– 80
21–60 "	70– 75
Old age	75– 80

In a female the pulse is quicker than in a male of the same age. The pulse is also quickened by excitement and after taking food, and is retarded by cold, sleep or fatigue.

In disease the pulse is slowed in certain ailments, such as kidney affections, and in certain injuries such as compression of the brain. It is quickened in many fevers, inflammatory affections and in debility.

To count the pulse place the fore, middle and ring fingers over the artery at the thumb-side of the wrist; count the beats for fifteen seconds, multiply this by four, and the result is the number of beats per minute.

Respiration—The number of average respirations per minute of an adult in good health is from sixteen to eighteen. In childhood it is higher.

The respiration can be counted by watching the movements of the chest, by listening to the breathing, or by placing the hands upon the chest and counting the number of movements per minute.

Bed-Sores—Bed-sores form on a weak or emaciated person about the hips, on the spine, shoulder blades, or wherever the bones press upon the flesh.

They should be treated when the first sign of redness or pain appears. The affected part should be bathed several times a day with alcohol and water. The pressure should be relieved by arranging pillows and placing the body upon them without allowing the affected place to touch anything. Air pillows can be procured for such a purpose. In absence of these, adhesive plaster strips may be applied in such a way as to relieve the pressure.

Apparent Death—Hold the hand of the person apparently dead before a candle or other light, the fingers stretched, one touching the other, and look through the space between the fingers toward the light. If the person is living, a red color will be seen where the fingers touch each other, due to the still circulating fluid blood as it shows itself between the transparent but yet congested tissues. When life is extinct this phenomenon ceases. Another method is to take a cold piece of polished steel, for instance a razor blade or table knife, and to hold this under the nose and before the mouth; if no moisture condenses upon it, it is safe to say that there is no breathing.

In cases of severe shock it is not sufficient to test the cessation of the heartbeat by feeling the pulse at the wrist. An acute ear can generally detect the movement of the heart by listening with the ear applied to the chest or back. Ordinarily it is very easy to decide between life and death, and the fear of being buried alive is without good foundation.

In cases of apparent death, it is best to disturb the patient as little as possible. Do not unnecessarily alarm friends, and do not give up working while there is the slightest ground for hope. The attendant should notice the exact time at which death takes place. Care should be taken not to announce death prematurely. Shortly after death, there may be a high rise of temperature, produced by chemical changes in the blood. This rise of temperature is followed by a peculiar stiffening of the muscles, called *rigor mortis*. Before this latter condition takes place, the body should be prepared for burial. If no undertaker is at hand, the body should be washed with a weak solution of some disinfectant.

If there is any difficulty in keeping the eyes shut, put a small wisp of cotton upon each eyeball under the lid. To keep the mouth closed, put a firm wedge under the jaw in the hollow of the throat. After the jaw is firmly set, the wedge may be removed. Straighten the legs by tying the feet together with a tape. Pack all the orifices of the body with absorbent cotton; bind a cloth around the hips. Over this any clothing desired may be adjusted. Cover the face and entire body with a sheet. Any slight discolorations may be made less conspicuous by dusting them with toilet powder.

After the removal of the body, the room should be thoroughly cleansed, all the appliances removed, the bedding and clothing sent out to be disinfected, and the room disinfected.

Feeding an Invalid—The kind of food to be given in every case should be decided by the physician; how to prepare and administer the food is a matter for the attendant. Everything should be the best of its kind, well cooked, seasoned and served. Food should never be prepared in the presence of an invalid, nor should the smell of cooking be allowed to reach him. The attendants should never eat in the sick room. Everything should be served as attractively as possible with clean napkins, spotless china, and shining silver and glass. Avoid spilling anything over the outside of dishes, or upon the tray, etc. Hot things should be served very hot, and cold things very cold. Bring everything into the sick room covered, either with dishes or napkins. Whatever is not eaten should at once be taken away; it is always better to bring too little than too much. Ascertain from the physician how much it is desirable that the patient should take in twenty-four hours, and divide the quantity up into portions suitable for regular intervals. As a rule the patient should never be aroused from sleep for food. Nourishment the last thing at night will often help to send the patient to sleep.

If the patient is helpless the attendant should assist by giving the food slowly, in small quantities, allowing each morsel to be swallowed before another is given. If there is difficulty in swallowing take advantage of the inspiration. In feeding a patient see that his head is not turned to either side, as this may cause the food to run out at the corner of the mouth instead of down the throat. Fluid food can be given conveniently through a bent glass tube, which is procurable at the drug stores.

In fevers there is often great thirst. Unless the physician advises to the contrary, it is safe to allow the patient all the water he may desire. It should be noted that a small glassful of water will be much more satisfactory than the same quantity in a larger vessel. Slightly bitter or acid drinks quench the thirst more fully than water alone. Hot water quenches thirst better than cold. Bits of ice are often refreshing. Small bits of ice swallowed whole or sips of very hot water are excellent to control vomiting.

EMERGENCY MEDICINES

It is not the intention of this Manual to encourage self-medication. In traveling, camping and on exploring expeditions, outfits of simple remedies for use in emergency are sometimes necessary (and in such cases it is recommended that a physician be consulted). It is particularly urged that a collection of drugs, and especially poisons, should not be kept in the household, factory or workshop, unless under lock and key, and in charge of a person skilled in their use.

The following articles are mentioned because they are often called for in emergencies and are more or less known in first aid practice:

Ammonia—It should be distinctly impressed upon the mind that there are several preparations of ammonia. All except aromatic spirit of ammonia are energetic preparations, highly irritating and poisonous if taken internally. Applied externally in any considerable strength, they cause blistering and pain. Ammonia in any form should not be applied to open wounds or irritated surfaces, except cautiously in the case of stings of insects, where the intention is to neutralize the poisons.

The vapor of the water of ammonia inhaled through the nostrils makes a powerful impression upon the nervous system, and is used in fainting and epilepsy, but it should be applied with caution. A strong preparation of ammonia applied to the nostrils is likely to produce a violent shock. A handkerchief or a wad of absorbent cotton or other material should be sprinkled with the ammonia and held at a safe distance from the nostrils. Contact with the skin will cause irritation. Water of ammonia is sometimes used in a diluted form, as an application for external pains, for mild chilblains and stings of insects. Combined with oils, it forms a very active liniment.

In purchasing ammonia water, the buyer should be cautious not to procure what is known as concentrated ammonia water.

Aromatic Spirit of Ammonia—This is the only preparation of ammonia intended for internal use. It is a stimulant, and is used in sick headache, hysteria, colic, or fainting, in doses from ten to thirty drops given in water.

Arnica—The tincture of arnica, sometimes called arnica liniment, is popularly supposed to be of value in accidents, especially those of the nature of sprains and bruises. It may not be generally known that arnica partakes of the nature of a poison, and is especially dangerous if taken internally. For external use strong preparations should not be applied full strength, as inflammation may follow in cases of tender skin.

Bicarbonate of Soda—Also known as baking soda. This preparation should be distinguished from sal soda or washing soda.

Bicarbonate of soda is used in the treatment of burns. It is also recommended as an antidote in poison by acids.

Camphor—Camphor is supplied by druggists in the form of gum camphor, or in liquid form in the shape of spirit or tincture of camphor. Its properties and uses are too well known to need comment. It should be remembered, however, that in large doses, when taken internally, camphor is a narcotic and irritant poison. It should never be taken in the solid form internally, except under the advice of

{116}

a physician. Spirit of camphor if given internally should be diluted with some other liquid, or dropped upon sugar. This course will prevent irritation of the mucous membrane of the mouth. The internal dose of the spirit of camphor is from one to twenty drops. Camphor should never be applied full strength directly to open wounds or to irritated or inflamed surfaces.

Ginger—The essence or tincture of ginger is a popular remedy, and is used in troubles of the digestive organs, bowel complaints, etc. The dose is from ten to forty drops in sweetened water, milk or other liquid.

Glycerine—Glycerine is sometimes recommended for burns. Mixed with equal parts of rosewater it makes a very soothing lotion for chapped hands.

Peppermint—The essence of peppermint or the tincture of peppermint is a well-known and popular remedy as an anti-spasmodic, a remedy in vomiting, colic and bowel complaints. The usual dose is from ten to twenty drops on sugar or in sweetened water. The oil of peppermint should not be used except under the advice of a physician.

Whisky—Whisky, brandy, wine and other spirits are by some considered necessary adjuncts to first aid. Their use is not recommended. Very often they do more harm than good. Hot water, coffee, tea or aromatic spirit of ammonia are to be preferred. When it is considered necessary to use alcoholic fluids, they should be of the very best quality, and should be used in small doses, in hot water, repeated if necessary. Children should never be given spirituous liquors except in extreme cases, where ten to twenty drops may be given in water.

Witch-Hazel—Known as extract of witch-hazel. This is a popular remedy for sprains, contusions, wounds and swellings. It forms a mild and suitable application for chapping, and is used by the laity for burns, scalds, cuts and abrasions. It has the merit of being non-irritating, and may with propriety be substituted for arnica, or the many highly irritating and dangerous liniments often recommended. It may be applied (full strengh or diluted with water) directly to the afflicted spot by the aid of a compress made of gauze or cloths saturated with the extract of witch-hazel.

Vaseline, Petrolatum, Albolene, Cosmoline, etc., are often recommended as applications for burns, scalds or inflammatory conditions. If of good quality, they are useful applications to a variety of injuries, being non-irritating and non-poisonous. They have also the merit of never becoming rancid, and are preferable to ointment or cold cream for emergency uses.

FORMULAS

Carron Oil—For burns and scalds. Mix equal parts of limewater and raw linseed oil; shake thoroughly. This forms a thick, cream-like emulsion that will keep almost indefinitely. Where burning accidents are frequent, this mixture should be kept on hand ready for use. It can be used freely, as no harm will arise from the application of any amount. If linseed oil is not at hand, olive oil or cotton seed oil may be used instead. Linseed oil is, however, the best.

ᵢ **Limewater**—Limewater may be procured ready made at any drug store, and the limewater obtained from reliable druggists is fit for both internal and external use. For external use in an emergency, where a drug store is not at hand, take a piece of lime weighing about one-half ounce (about the size of a walnut), slake it by gradually pouring water over it in small portions at a time. When slaked put in a bottle or other vessel and pour on a quart of water (cold); let it stand; pour off as wanted for use. In an emergency it may be used at once without clarifying.

Be Prepared

True efficiency in the application of First Aid means that whenever and wherever an emergency occurs there is a person at hand ready to meet it. Preparedness in First Aid means a knowledge of what to do, and doing the right thing at the right time.

Being prepared implies the having at hand the means and the things needed for the application of First Aid. Large industries, mines, service corporations and factories have installed elaborate emergency equipment and systems for ready application of First Aid Measures. The shop, the store, the home, the auto car, the traveler and even the individual should have at hand suitable supplies for the emergency applications of First Aid.

To be ready to at once apply first aid in emergency means the saving of life and limb, the avoidance of pain and suffering, the saving of money through loss of time and wages and the outgo consequent upon illness that might have been avoided through preparedness. To be prepared to apply First Aid in emergency to one's self, to one's family, or to a fellow man, is one of the highest duties of modern life.

COMMUNICABLE DISEASES

CLOSELY allied to first aid, indeed now considered a legitimate part of a first aid system, is a knowledge of measures to prevent the spread of communicable disease.

Sanitation, hygiene, the prevention of sickness and death are within the realm of the first aid worker.

Communicable diseases*—also called contagious or infectious diseases—are spread by means of microscopic bodies called germs, passing from person to person directly, or by means of discharges called secretions or excretions.

These germs are so small that millions of them unperceived may gain entrance to the body through the throat, nose and skin. In vigorous health their presence may do no harm, as they are not likely to find a soil suitable to their growth, but in failing health, as in weakness, in a slight cold, inflammation or depressed vitality, a place is found where they can lodge, grow and multiply. Secreted upon or excreted from the diseased body they are carried from person to person.

They cling to cloths, clothing, bedding, carpets and to the hair and skin of animals. They find their way into food, milk, meats, fruits; they may be carried on the bodies of insects. Persons and things may become carriers of the seeds of disease.

The most effective means for the control, prevention and ultimate eradication of communicable diseases are: isolation (the separation of the sick from the well); disinfection (destruction of infection), and in the case of smallpox, diphtheria, and certain other diseases, vaccination.

The suggestions which follow are intended to be used while awaiting specific instructions from the attending physician, and as supplemental to his instruction. They only include measures tending to prevent the spread of the disease. The treatment of the patient should always be carried out by a physician. These suggestions embrace a condensed resumé of methods endorsed by authorities. They are purposely brief and are adapted to ordinary conditions.

Local or State Boards of Health publish rules governing the control of communicable disease. These rules should be followed.

How to Avoid Contagious Diseases

Avoid sitting down in the sick room as much as possible. Especially avoid sitting on the bed. Do not even lean against the bed, walls or furniture.

*COMMUNICABLE DISEASES—Formerly the term "contagious" was applied to certain diseases supposed to be spread by direct or indirect contact, and the term "infectious" was applied to disease supposed to be transferred in an indirect manner. Under our present idea these terms are inaccurate and confusing, the more correct term being communicable (or transmissible), which means that the disease in question may be communicable from one person to another or in some instances from animal to man.

Wash the hands with antiseptic soap after each contact with the patient.

Exercise regularly, if possible in the open air.

Nurses and persons attending the sick should wear washable dresses, which should be changed frequently. A washable cap should cover the hair.

Keep so far from a sick person that his breath will not reach you directly. Above all avoid kissing or whispering.

Do not put to your lips any food, drink, dish or utensil that the patient has touched, or that has been in the sick room.

Do not eat or drink in the sick room.

Wear no clothing that the patient has worn just before, during, or just after his sickness.

Keep the hands free from all discharges from the sick. If the hands are accidentally contaminated, wash them at once with an antiseptic soap.

If the patient be sick with any of the eruptive diseases, such as smallpox or scarlet fever, take every precaution not to come in contact with the scales or scabs of the skin.

Kill or drive out of the sick room all flies or other insects. Be sure to destroy all mosquitoes.

THE SICK ROOM

Select a large, airy, light and pleasant room. It should be as quiet as possible.

Before the room is occupied by the patient, it should be made bare of hangings, carpets and upholstery. Unnecessary articles of furniture should be removed. A light iron bedstead, one chair and a table are sufficient.

Clean the walls and woodwork by wiping with a wet cloth before bringing in the patient.

Keep the room always at a temperature of seventy degrees.

Avoid all sweeping. Depend upon scrubbing for cleansing the floor.

Avoid dusting with a brush. Use cloths dampened with a disinfectant solution for walls and furniture.

Keep the room always aired and at a temperature as nearly even as possible.

Let in all the direct sunlight possible, unless it seems to hurt the patient's eyes.

Bedding should be changed frequently. Throw the soiled bed clothes into a tub or pail containing a disinfecting solution.

Towels, napkins, or bandages should always be clean. They should be taken from the room and disinfected after each time of using.

All dishes, cups, glasses, spoons, and utensils which have been in the sick room should be disinfected before being taken out. Scalding hot water and soap are effective for this purpose.

Toys, shears, vases, combs, brushes or anything that has come near the patient should be disinfected or destroyed.

It is a good rule in communicable diseases to consider that everything that has been carried into the sick room has become infected and needs disinfecting before being used elsewhere.

Dishes used by the patient should not be used by others until cleansed, or washed with other dishes.

The food should be brought into the room just before the patient is ready for it. All articles of food left should be burned, or else mixed with a disinfectant and buried. Do not allow milk or other food to stand in the sick room. Whatever drink or food has been in the room, must not be used by others, or fed to animals.

The bodily discharges from the sick should all be considered dangerous. In typhoid fever, the bodily excreta is the ordinary means of infection. The eruptions of some diseases, though ordinarily supposed to appear only on the surface of the skin, are equally common inside the body, throughout the whole alimentary canal. Therefore in all the dangerous diseases care must be taken to avoid infection from the discharges. Discharges must be considered to include sputum as well, for the sputum is the source of infection in tuberculosis, diphtheria, and other maladies.

Excreta from the bowels or kidneys should immediately be covered with a disinfectant solution. The vessel containing the discharges and disinfectants should be shaken and after half an hour the contents thrown into the watercloset, or if there be no closet with sewer connection, buried in the ground. The discharges should never be thrown where they might contaminate a running stream. Vessels used to catch discharges should be thoroughly disinfected with boiling water and a disinfectant.

CHICKEN-POX

This is a specific infectious disease of childhood. The appearance of an eruption marks the beginning of the disease. The eruption usually appears first in the trunk, then spreads to the face and the rest of the body. It is well marked on the scalp. A group of small, red spots develops and within twenty-four hours become capped with clear, tear-drop vesicles. The vesicles develop in crops. Take ordinary hygienic measures and keep the patient in bed. Prevent scratching, as the vesicle often results in a scar. Children should not be sent to school or allowed to mingle with other children for at least two weeks after the recovery of the last one affected in the home. A doctor should be summoned, the so-called chicken-pox may be smallpox.

TUBERCULOSIS

Tuberculosis, otherwise known as phthisis or consumption, is a germ disease and is conveyed from one person to another by means of the spittle. Tuberculosis of the lungs is very insidious, and if neglected usually proves fatal.

The first indications often suggest a lowering of vitality, rather than any specific disease. There may be a poor appetite, gradual loss of weight, lassitude or weakness and indisposition to exertion, sensitiveness to cold, palpitation of the heart, slight fever, especially in the afternoon or evening, indigestion, neuralgic pains, slight cough or clearing of the throat in the morning, and lingering colds. It is very important that one who experiences the slight symptoms which are the first warning of tuberculosis should at once place himself under the care of a competent physician without trying to treat himself, or waiting for more alarming symptoms to appear.

A tuberculous person should not expect to be cured by medicine, but by persistent effort on his part, and by faithfully following the directions of his physician.

Since the sputum is by far the most important, if not the sole means by which the germs are cast off from the patient's body, there is practically no danger from tuberculous persons who take proper care of the sputum instead of expectorating promiscuously, and such care is to be insisted upon and encouraged by every possible means.

There is nothing more necessary for a person having tuberculosis than the constant use of a sputum cup. He should spit nowhere except into an antiseptic sputum cup.

The following simple rules should be enforced in every case of tuberculosis:

Never cough without a handkerchief before your mouth; it endangers others. Never cough in a dining-room. Never swallow your expectoration, or cough while lying on your back. Thoroughly cleanse the mouth before eating. All sputum must be destroyed. Do not expectorate on the ground, supposing that the sun's rays will thoroughly disinfect the sputum. Such a belief is erroneous and pernicious. All persons who cough should refrain from kissing. The patient who conscientiously carries out these simple precautions is not a menace to those about him.

His room and his clothing should be disinfected occasionally. In case of his removal from one house to another, or upon his death, the house (especially his own apartment) should be thoroughly disinfected before being occupied by others.

Those having tuberculosis are warned against the many widely advertised cures, specifics and special methods of treatment of consumption. No cure can be expected from any kind of treatment except the regularly accepted method known to every reputable physician. This treatment depends for its success upon pure air, sunshine, outdoor life and nourishing food. Rest, both physical and mental, is an important factor in the treatment. An *early* diagnosis by a physician is particularly important.

COLDS

Colds are contagious; they are caused by germs.

The germs are spread through the discharges from the mouth and throat from one person to another.

Draughts, wet feet, sudden changes of the temperature do not cause colds. These conditions, however, weaken the body and favor the growth of germs and the development of the cold. If neglected, colds may be complicated by diseases of the ears and sinuses. Pneumonia may be a serious outcome. In children, a persistent discharge from the nose may be due to enlarged and infected adenoids.

Preventive Rules for Colds—Do not get close to others who have colds.

Do not use handkerchiefs, towels or cups that have been used by people who have colds.

Do not sneeze or cough except into your own handkerchief.

Do not spit on the floor, and thus spread colds, tuberculosis and other diseases.

Do not neglect a cold. During the first few days if you have fever stay in bed. This will help you and protect others from getting your cold. Take a laxative and use simple household remedies. If these do not help you, call a doctor.

Keep your body in good condition and your resistance to the germs causing colds will be increased.

DIPHTHERIA

Diphtheria is now known to be a preventable disease. If every baby and child be given suitable injections of Toxin-Anti-Toxin, diphtheria will become as rare as smallpox. To make sure that the Toxin-Anti-Toxin has immunized the child against diphtheria, a Shick Test should be performed. Consult your doctor about these inoculations.

Diphtheria is principally a children's disease, although grown persons are by no means safe from its ravages.

On the slightest suspicion of sore throat, especially among children, a physician should be summoned. The child should immediately be separated from all other persons, except necessary attendants.

Every person known to be sick with diphtheria should be promptly and completely isolated from the public. Only such attendants as are actually necessary should have charge of or visit the patient, and these should be restricted in their intercourse with other persons.

Since the special contagion of diphtheria is in the mouth, nose and throat, the greatest care must be taken of the discharges. It is best to receive it in a spit-cup or spittoon containing a disinfectant, or upon cloths to be burned. Clothing, towels, bed linen, or any clothes that have come in contact with the patient should, before removal from the sick room, be placed in a pail or tub of water containing a disinfectant, then boiled in water.

Nurses and attendants should have at hand a disinfectant soap for washing the hands and face when about to leave the sick room, or for washing the hands after each contact with the patient.

All patients who have had diphtheria must remain quietly in bed for two or three weeks after all symptoms have disappeared.

Before persons who have had diphtheria are allowed to associate with others, two or more successive negative throat cultures should be obtained by the physician.

At the time of an epidemic of diphtheria, rooms which have been occupied by a patient should be thoroughly disinfected. School children should be carefully watched and any case of sore throat or other suspicious symptoms reported. School children should be cautioned against the use of common drinking cups, the exchange of pencils, books and chewing gum. Permit no child in whose family diphtheria exists to attend school.

The greatest advance in the treatment of diphtheria has been the discovery of anti-toxin. A sufficient dose should be administered by a physician without delay. In illness of any severity which is suspected of being diphtheria, and in croup, it is far better for the doctor to administer the treatment at once, than to delay the treatment until a diagnosis has been made.

Children who have been exposed to infection should be immunized with prophylactic doses of anti-toxin without delay. Consult your doctor.

Rules for Avoiding Diphtheria

Even the mildest case of diphtheria is dangerous.

Do not let a child go near a case of diphtheria.

Do not allow a dog, cat or other animal to enter the sick room.

Allow no person to visit the sick room.

Wear or handle no clothing from a sick room.

Use no dish used by the sick. Allow no child to use any dishes or toys that have been in the sick room unless they have been thoroughly disinfected.

In epidemics regard all persons having sore throat as probable diphtheria patients. Never kiss such persons, and observe all care about allowing children to touch their clothes or dishes. Keep your children away from them as much as possible.

After a death or recovery from diphtheria, the room in which there has been a case should, with all its contents, be thoroughly disinfected. As the dead body of a diphtheria patient is extremely dangerous, the interment should be as soon as possible. Public funerals in case of diphtheria should not be permitted.

MEASLES

Measles is one of the eruptive fevers, usually recognized by its peculiar catarrhal symptoms and the characteristic rash.

As the germ or germs of measles are easily transmitted, the separation of the sick from the well is necessary and should be strict.

The patient should be kept from school until recovery is complete.

The prevention of the spread of measles depends for success upon two things—keeping the sick from contact with the well (isolation), and cleanliness in respect to the things handled by the sick.

Because of the serious complications that may follow, it is always advisable to have a physician in attendance.

Quarantine regulations in measles should be continued for two weeks after the appearance of the last case in the household.

The disease is transferable for some time before it is recognized. Therefore parents should learn to treat all "colds" in children as suspicious, and to guard against contact with other children until the nature of the cold is ascertained.

German Measles—Of this disease but little is known. It is the general opinion that it is less communicable than the ordinary measles or scarlet fever, with either of which it may be confounded. The first and generally the only symptoms are some catarrh and slight fever. Quarantine is not necessary. It is wise, however, to keep children in whose family there are cases of German measles from school for a week or ten days, as many cases supposed to be German measles are really cases of scarlet fever. A physician should be consulted when the first symptoms appear.

CEREBROSPINAL FEVER

This disease is variously called also by the names spinal meningitis, cerebral meningitis, acute meningitis, infectious meningitis, cerebrospinal meningitis, spinal fever and spotted fever.

Children and young adults are the most susceptible. Meningitis is a communicable disease. It is believed that meningitis is spread through the discharges from the nose and throat.

There is obtainable a curative serum, known as anti-meningitis serum. Consult your doctor.

Isolation and disinfection are means which should be employed to prevent the spread of the disease. Particular attention should be given to discharges from the throat and nose.

In times of epidemics every case of cold should receive attention, and young persons should be kept from crowded places. Personal cleanliness, especially of the mouth, throat and nose, should have more than usual care.

INFANTILE PARALYSIS

This is primarily a disease of childhood but no age is immune. In recent years epidemics have occurred with increasing frequency. While little is known as to the methods by which infantile paralysis is transmitted, it has been established that the virus or the germ of the disease is present in the discharges from the nose, throat, and bowels of those ill with the disease.

It has been claimed, but not proven, that the virus may be transmitted by the bite of certain species of flies. It has also been suggested that the disease may be conveyed by dust, contaminated foods, and by inoculation through wounds.

Experienced physicians are at times puzzled in making an accurate diagnosis of infantile paralysis, hence it would be quite futile for a layman to make an attempt.

At times when the disease is prevalent in a community symptoms which should be regarded as suspicious are fever, vomiting, diarrhea, listlessness, unusual fretfulness and drowsiness. When one or more of these symptoms appear a physician should be called at once.

ᵗ Patients with infantile paralysis must be isolated for a period of from six to eight weeks.

Children who have been exposed to the disease should be isolated for a period of at least two weeks, and adults should be kept under observation for a like length of time.

The sick room should be effectually screened and household pets should be excluded.

So far as is known the essence of the prevention of the spread of the disease is to maintain conditions of rigid cleanliness.

The cloths used to receive the discharges from the mouth and nose of the patient should be burned.

The discharges from the bowels should be disinfected.

It is perhaps unnecessary to urge that in times when this disease is epidemic the assembling of children either at play or in other gatherings should be discontinued. In some instances it is necessary to close the schools.

Children in families where there is infantile paralysis should not be allowed to leave their homes.

MUMPS

Children between the ages of four and fourteen are most susceptible. The disease is contagious from the beginning of the symptoms and for several days after the swelling has disappeared. It is conveyed by contact or through the spittle. The characteristic symptoms are swelling of the face just in front of or below the angle of the jaw. Chewing becomes painful and at times there is fever, headache, vomiting, and general depression. The patient should be quarantined for three weeks and no children should be allowed to return to school or to mingle with other children for at least twenty days after the last case of the disease in the household. The complications of this disease are more dangerous than the disease itself.

During the attack, rest in bed is essential.

PINK EYE

This disease is conveyed by the discharges from the affected eye. There is pain, headache and sensitiveness to the light. There is a great tendency to transmission in the use of a common hand towel, or in the lending of a handkerchief. Children afflicted with pink eye should not be allowed to mingle with other children or be sent to school. All articles used by the patient should be carefully disinfected, boiling water being sufficient in this case. All cases of inflammation of the eye should be treated by a physician.

RINGWORM

This disease is easily communicated. It flourishes particularly among those who are dirty and neglected, but it may attack children who receive the best of care. Ringworm is recognized by its peculiar scabby sore or patch. It may occur upon the face or other parts of the body, but most frequently it attacks the scalp where it produces bald areas on which are stubby growths of broken and diseased hair. It is often very persistent and may resist treatment for many months. A physician should be consulted immediately upon the appearance of a case of ringworm. Under proper treatment a child need not be excluded from school. Care should be taken to avoid the exchange of wearing apparel, particularly hats, and to prevent close contact with the person afflicted.

Persons having ringworm should use separate towels, soaps and other toilet utensils. Toilet articles used by them should be boiled after each use.

SCABIES

This disease is transferred by close contact. It is accompanied by roughness and cracking of the skin, with severe itching, which is usually worse at night. The skin at the base of and between the fingers is especially liable to be affected, although the entire body may be involved. Children with itch should not attend school, or mingle with other children, unless they are being treated by a physician. At times when this disease is prevalent the children should be instructed as to the nature of the disease, and cautioned against wearing the clothes of others, such as hats, gloves, or baseball mitts. They should not be allowed to take hold of hands in games, or to use books in common with others. Persons afflicted with itch should use separate towels, soap and other toilet articles.

SCARLET FEVER

Scarlet Fever is an acute infectious disease, characterized by a sore throat, a rash on the skin and roof of the mouth, followed by desquamation (peeling of the skin).

In most cases infection occurs by direct contact. It may also be communicated indirectly, although infrequently, by articles contaminated by the germ. It can likewise be conveyed by milk that has become infected by handling.

The period during which the patient can transmit the disease is indefinite. It is probable that scarlet fever is not communicable during the period of incubation, and that it is only slightly so during the onset of the disease. In the past, the period of peeling has been considered the infectious time; but this is no longer considered true. Probably the infection is carried from persistent discharges from the nose, ears and throat. Their presence should determine the length of quarantine. In mild cases, when discharges from the upper respiratory tract are absent, from three to four weeks isolation should be sufficient.

The onset of scarlet fever is usually very abrupt. A child may seem perfectly well and suddenly become ill with nausea, fever, and sore throat. Vomiting is one of the most constant early symptoms. Although the face is flushed, there is no definite rash until six to twenty-four hours later. The rash usually appears first on the neck, behind the ears, and on the chest, gradually spreading within twenty-four hours to the arms and legs, and then quite uniformly over the entire surface of the body. Various complications particularly of the ears and kidneys can occur, and should be carefully watched for by the physician.

Susceptible people may be immunized by the injection of scarlet fever streptococcus toxin. The degree and length of the immunity has not as yet been satisfactorily ascertained, though it seems to last at least one year.

Children or others exposed to scarlet fever should be watched closely for sore throat or other symptoms of the disease, and the temperature taken twice daily.

TYPHOID FEVER

Typhoid, or enteric, fever is a most severe disease of the intestines to which persons of all ages are liable.

The greatest number of deaths from typhoid fever occur in persons in the prime of life. A person having this disease in a mild form may impart it in a fatal form to another.

The germ, or seed, of typhoid fever enters the body through the mouth and attacks the walls of the small intestines. The poison produced by the germ in the course of its growth gives rise to the typhoid inflammation.

The discharges from the sick, such as the stools, urine and sputum, carry the infective agent. These discharges easily reach and contaminate food, water and milk, and in this way the disease is spread from the sick to the well.

Infected water, milk, uncooked green vegetables, contaminated with infected water or soil, uncooked oysters and shell-fish from polluted water have been known to be a source of the disease.

Flies and other insects feed and breed upon the infected discharges of typhoid patients and carry infection to the food supply of the well.

Persons living in the same house, or who visit a typhoid patient, may carry away the germs of typhoid on their hands or clothing, and by these and other means the infection may be transmitted.

The symptoms of typhoid fever are at times very obscure. Some of the symptoms are described as vomiting, depression and the slow onset of fever.

In times when typhoid fever is present in a community, or at any time when symptoms of this character are present, a competent physician should be called at once. The symptoms may manifest themselves in from one to four weeks after exposure to the infection.

At times persons may carry typhoid fever ("walking" cases, "carriers") without being troubled with any of the severer manifestations of the disease, but such mild cases may transfer the disease in its most virulent form.

Typhoid fever is communicable from the sick to the well from the beginning of the disease for an indefinite period.

Sedgwick, an eminent authority, has stated that in the prevention of typhoid fever the problem is "to keep the excreta of A (the patient) out of the mouth of B (the well)."

The measures which will tend to prevent the spread of this disease are as follows:

The reporting of the disease to the health authorities.

The early diagnosis of the disease, for which purpose what is known as bacteriological diagnosis may be carried out through a local or state laboratory.

The sick should be separated from the well. If proper isolation cannot be secured the patient should be taken to a hospital.

The discharges from the sick should be carefully disinfected.

The sputum should be collected and destroyed as in tuberculosis.

Isolation should not be terminated until the patient's discharges are free from germs, which can be determined only by laboratory examination.

The prevention of the pollution and infection of water and food supplies, especially milk, is an important part in the control of typhoid fever.

Protective inoculation against typhoid fever has been employed, and anti-typhoid fever vaccine has been used to a limited extent in communities to prevent the spread of epidemics.

At times when typhoid fever is prevalent in a community or neighborhood, or when present in the household, the following measures should be observed:

For drinking purposes use only water known to be pure, or water which has been boiled.

All milk, the source of which is not absolutely free from suspicion, should be brought to the boiling point.

Raw shell-fish, such as oysters, should not be eaten. Cooking destroys the germs.

Avoid green fruit and other things liable to set up indigestion and diarrhea.

Avoid bathing at beaches or in rivers or lakes near the opening of a sewer.

See that windows and doors are protected by fly screens, especially those of kitchen and dining room.

Every case of diarrhea is to be suspected, and should be treated as a case of typhoid. All decaying animal and vegetable matter around any premises should be removed, and both it and the drains, vaults, and damp places thoroughly disinfected.

Disinfect all manure piles and privy vaults in order to destroy flies.

Do not visit the sick room unless it is absolutely necessary.

Do not eat or drink anything that has been in any way connected with a typhoid patient.

DYSENTERIC DISEASES

Dysentery and diarrhea are now considered communicable or transferable in the same way as typhoid fever. Certain of these diseases may become epidemic and may be spread through a community as is the case with typhoid.

Some forms of dysentery are known to be caused by germs, others are of unknown or obscure origin.

All forms of dysentery should be cared for in the same manner as outlined for typhoid fever.

Cases should be placed in the care of a physician at once, the patient isolated, and discharges disinfected.

Flies should be guarded against. General measures of thorough cleanliness and disinfection should be established.

SMALLPOX

This disease is also known as varioloid, or variola, and sometimes erroneously called Puerto Rican chicken-pox.

Smallpox is one of the most easily communicated and dangerous of diseases. The contagion of smallpox may be carried from one person to another by actual contact, or it may be carried from place to place by means of infected clothing, bedding, merchandise, letters, or any other infected article.

Smallpox is a preventable disease. Upon the first appearance of a case in any locality, systematic vaccination should be resorted to. In times of epidemic, revaccination should follow in all cases where the operation has not been successfully performed within the preceding twelve months. Vaccination should in all cases be performed by a qualified physician. Smallpox in any form requires strict methods of quarantine and disinfection. Every case of suspected smallpox should be reported at once to the local board of health.

WHOOPING COUGH

Whooping cough is primarily a children's disease, cases in persons above ten years of age being rare.

The germ of whooping cough finds a lodgment in the throat and is scattered through the air by the coughing of the sufferer. This disease is easily conveyed from one child to another.

Whooping cough usually passes through three stages. The first stage lasts about ten days and can hardly be distinguished from an ordinary cold. The spasmodic stage lasts about one month and is accompanied by the characteristic whoop. The last stage often lingers for months, especially during the winter. The unmistakable symptom is the spasmodic cough followed by the crowing sound, usually accompanied by the expulsion of a thick mucus and sometimes by vomiting, and bleeding at the nose. Whooping cough patients should be quarantined for about six weeks, or until the end of the spasmodic coughing. Children should not be allowed to attend school if there is a case of whooping cough in the family.

The early use of vaccines is sometimes found beneficial.

A child with whooping cough should be kept separate from all other children. The sputum should be received in sputum cups or vessels containing a disinfectant, or on cloths or paper handkerchiefs that can be burned. After recovery the patient's clothing should be disinfected.

COMMUNICABLE DISEASES OF ANIMALS

Many diseases of animals are more or less communicable to man as well as to other animals. Among these are the following: glanders, lumpy jaw, nasal gleet, scab in sheep, anthrax, epizootic.

When any of these diseases are present or suspected, all harness, bits, blankets and covers should be disinfected by washing with hot water and a disinfectant. Straw and anything else used in bedding should be burned. The walls of the stable should be washed with a strong solution of a disinfectant and hot water. This should be repeated until recovery or death of the animal.

Afterwards go over the stable, washing thoroughly with the disinfectant, burning up all rubbish until the barn is safe.

All well animals should be kept in a clean, fresh place.

INSECTS AS CARRIERS OF DISEASE

It has been established that many diseases, including malarial fever, yellow fever, typhoid fever, scarlet fever and smallpox are carried by insects, such as mosquitoes and flies.

It has been found that measures directed against certain insects have been the means of stamping out or at least of assisting to eradicate infection. In every communicable disease, it would therefore seem a wise precaution to kill all mosquitoes and other insects around the sick room; to prevent insects from biting both the persons who are sick, and those who are well; to prevent insects from having access to the sick room or from coming in contact with food intended for persons who are well.

Doors and windows should be screened in neighborhoods where contagious diseases may be carried by insects.

It is known that mosquitoes breed in pools of water and in damp places. All pools should be drained or filled; all cans, barrels, or other receptacles for the collection of water should be cleaned out. In case filling or draining is not possible, the places should be freely sprinkled with a disinfectant or kerosene oil.

FUMIGATION

Where it is desired to fumigate a room after recovery or death from infectious disease, it is necessary to understand how to go about the matter in a way that will accomplish the result.

Fumigation by means of formaldehyd gas has largely displaced the use of sulphur for this purpose.

All articles in the room that can be spared had better be burned.

Preparation for fumigation should be made as follows:

In all rooms to be disinfected, cupboards, drawers and closets should be opened; clothing and bedding should be hung upon ropes or over chairs or other furniture. Unroll all window shades. Spread everything out in as thin layers as possible.

The reason for this is that formaldehyd gas has but little penetrating power and hence all articles of clothing and bedding must be spread out or hung up so that the gas can come into contact with as much material as possible.

Cracks of windows and doors should be stuffed with cloths or paper or sealed with adhesive plaster. Close all openings of every kind with paper or cloth. The success of disinfection depends upon the care with which the rooms are sealed.

Except in warm humid weather it is advisable to sprinkle water upon the floor or hang a wet sheet on a rope stretched across the room. This is done to increase the humidity and make the disinfection more thorough.

The room to be disinfected should always be warm. Above 70 degrees Fahrenheit is advisable.

Formaldehyd gas will not kill the germs unless it is used in sufficient quantity and under proper conditions.

Formaldehyd gas does not damage anything in the household and is not poisonous to man or beast, unless it is inhaled in very large quantities. It will not destroy flies, mosquitoes, bedbugs and the like.

The rapidity with which the gas is given off is an important factor. If the leakage is extensive and the generation of the gas is slow, the amount of gas in the room at any one period of time may be less than sufficient.

After starting the fumigator the operator should leave the room, close the door tightly behind him, seal the cracks, and allow it to remain closed for from four to six hours or, better still, over night. Then open the room, airing it thoroughly until little or no fumes of formaldehyd gas can be detected by the eyes and nose.

For fumigation purposes either the liquid formaldehyd, also called formalin, or the dry solid paraformaldehyd, also called paraform, may be used, but on account of the troublesomeness of all methods of using the liquid, most forms of fumigators purchasable at the stores contain the dry paraform.

According to Bulletins of the United States Public Health Service, it is advisable to use not less than two ounces of paraform for every one thousand cubic feet of space in the room to be disinfected. It does no harm to use more.

Therefore, before purchasing fumigators, it is necessary to measure roughly the room and calculate in the following manner: Let us say the room measures 12 feet long, 10 feet wide and 8 feet high. Multiply 12 x 10 x 8 and we get 960 cubic feet. As most of the commercial fumigators are made up in 1-ounce, 2-ounce and 4-ounce sizes, it will be satisfactory to select the 2-ounce size for the above room.

To Prevent the Spread of Disease

Call a physician when the first symptoms appear.

Keep the sick from contact with the well. (Isolation.)

Cleanse and disinfect all things that have come in contact with the sick.

When the physician shall advise, use vaccination, injection of serums, etc.

Keep flies and insects from the sick room.

Keep household pets away from the sick.

Disinfect the bodily discharges of the sick, especially the sputum.

In water borne diseases boil and cool drinking water.

Do not neglect colds. Colds are communicable. They are often the beginning of serious diseases.

Watch mild cases of diphtheria, measles, scarlet fever, and like maladies. They may produce virulent cases in others.

Consider the period of recovery dangerous. In many diseases the apparently well may still convey the disease.

Keep sick children from school until the doctor advises their return. After recovery or death cleanse and disinfect clothing and premises.

FIRST AID OUTFITS

THE prompt application of first aid has been made possible through the assembling of essential first aid dressings in compact cases. Manufacturers of surgical dressings have devised a series of first aid outfits suitable for use in industries, in shops, in schools and public buildings and in homes. They also offer outfits especially designed to be carried in automobiles, in traveling bags and even in the vest pocket or the lady's handbag.

Without proper dressings at hand the first aid worker is seriously handicapped. It is now known that the greatest danger from wounds is infection. A wound is easily contaminated by contact with the bacteria-laden air, clothing, or unclean dressings, possibly resulting in blood-poisoning, gangrene, inflammation, fever, erysipelas, lockjaw or tetanus, and a train of other complications.

It is very important, in first aid, that all dressings applied to a wound shall not only look clean, but shall be surgically clean (aseptic), that is, free from infection or surgical dirt.

With a first aid outfit at hand, a first aid worker is always prepared to instantly apply a surgically clean dressing of the best type.

The various outfits now available are so arranged and the contents are so selected that temporary aid can be rendered by any layman, and when the physician arrives he will find proper material at hand for his use.

Some of the first aid outfits designed and supplied by the publishers of this Manual are described on the following pages. These outfits are sold through drug stores in all parts of the country. The contents of these outfits are all standard articles and can be replaced as soon as used, through your drug store, thus making possible a fully stocked outfit at all times.

JOHNSON'S FIRST AID CABINET No. 1

Many thousands of this type of cabinet have been installed in industrial establishments, public schools, municipal departments, offices, steamships, transportation lines and construction projects.

It contains ample supplies and will fulfill every requirement, excepting in those States where special enactments call for certain items not contained in these cabinets, which conditions are met in Johnson's First Aid Cabinet, No. 10.

The Cabinet is made of heavy decorated japanned metal, with strong hinges, fasteners and hangers, and convenient handles for carrying.

The dressings and supplies are packed in separate metal compartments with the contents of each compartment plainly printed on the

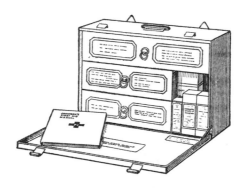

outside. This system automatically keeps every thing in its place. The cabinet solves a problem that has for some time confronted first aid workers in industrial plants—protection from factory dust and dirt. The outside metal door, the metal compartments and the dust-proof wrappers of the packages themselves, throw a triple protection around the dressings and supplies. The importance which first aid authorities place in the absolute cleanliness of first aid dressings, gives this feature special significance.

In each cabinet there is extra space for additional dressings of the type most needed in the particular occupation.

CONTENTS

Absorbent Gauze
Absorbent Cotton
"ZO" Adhesive Plaster
Cotton Roller Bandages
Linton Gauze Bandages
Johnson's First Aid for Wounds Packet No. 3
Picric Acid Gauze Pads
Applicator Sticks wound with cotton
Finger Cots (assorted sizes)
Esmarch Triangular Bandage
Aromatic Spirit of Ammonia
Carbolized Petrolatum
Camphenol. Empty bottle for Camphenol Solution
Alcoholic Solution of Iodine
Wooden Splints. Tourniquet
Band-Aid
Safety Pins
Scissors. Tweezers
Johnson's Standard First Aid Manual
Blanks for reporting accidents
Blanks for inventory and ordering refill supplies

JOHNSON'S FIRST AID CABINET No. 10

This cabinet is a variation or modification of Cabinet No. 1, devised to meet the specifications of the New York State statute. It complies with the Compensation Board requirements of nearly every State in the Union. It more than meets the specifications of the companies working under the title "Compensation Rating and Accident Board," which issues insurance under the compensation laws of the various States. In fact, this cabinet contains a much larger supply of material than any of the Board lists specify, making it possible to take care of a great number of cases before the necessity of replenishment arises. The containing case is of the same type as the No. 1 Cabinet.

CONTENTS

First Aid for Wounds Packet
Absorbent Gauze
Absorbent Cotton
"ZO" Adhesive Plaster
Cotton Roller Bandages
Lintor. Gauze Bandages
Picric Acid Gauze Pads
Finger Cots (assorted sizes)
Esmarch Triangular Bandage
Aromatic Spirit of Ammonia
Camphenol disinfectant
Bicarbonate of Soda and Petrolatum 3%
Boric Acid Solution 4%
Alcoholic Solution of Iodine
Castor Oil
Band-Aid
Wooden Applicators wound with cotton
Wooden Tongue Depressors
Medicine Glass
Wooden Splints
Tourniquet
Scissors; Tweezers
Safety Pins
Johnson's Standard First Aid Manual
Blanks for reporting accidents
Blanks for inventory and ordering refill supplies

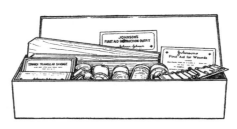

WOOD'S EMERGENCY CASE No. 6

This case is designed for camp, summer bungalow, automobile, launch, home, or small shop, where a compact and convenient accident outfit is desired. It contains material applicable to large and small injuries, and a book of instruction. The case is of japanned metal, with hinged cover and fastener.

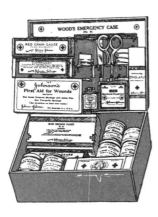

CONTENTS

First Aid for Wounds Packet No. 3
Burn Dressing Packet No. 22
Absorbent Gauze (Red Cross)
Absorbent Cotton
Linton Gauze Bandages
Cotton Bandages
"ZO" Adhesive Plaster
Carbolized Petrolatum
Tourniquet
Alcoholic Solution of Iodine
Band-Aid
Scissors. Tweezers
Safety Pins
Handbook of First Aid

JOHNSON'S HOUSEKIT

The Housekit is designed especially for the home. Beauty and utility are combined—complete first aid protection is packed into a cabinet that is worthy of a place in the home. The metal case, decorated in gray enamel, is designed to hang upon the wall —the door lowering to form a shelf.

It contains material especially selected to meet emergencies liable to arise in the home, and a handbook of instructions.

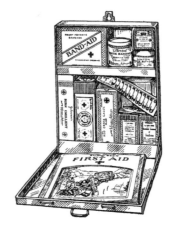

AUTOKIT No. 8

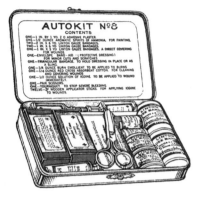

The constant increase in highway travel has made first aid protection for the motorist a necessity. State and Federal authorities are urging that every automobile be equipped with a first aid kit.

The Autokit is especially designed for the automobile. It can be carried in the car pocket or under the seat, a canvas jacket protecting the decorated metal case.

The Autokit contains material suitable for the care of ordinary injuries which may occur in the garage or on the road, and a book of instruction. The motorist who carries an Autokit can render first aid in a simple and effective manner, giving relief and protection in accidents liable to happen miles from a doctor or a hospital.

JOHNSON'S TRAVELKIT

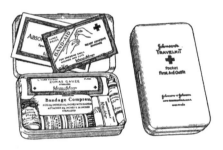

This is a pocket-size, light metal case, containing first aid supplies necessary to take care of emergencies while traveling.

It has been adopted by sportsmen, campers, Boy and Girl Scouts and vacationists. It can conveniently be carried in the pocket, in a traveling bag or in the side pocket of an automobile. Its substantial metal case will stand long usage. A book of instruction is packed in every case.

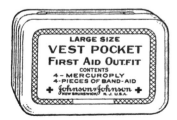

VEST POCKET OUTFIT

This outfit is small enough to carry in the vest pocket, lady's handbag, or child's pocket. It enables a person to instantly dress any small injury and thus prevent infection. Contains four Mercuroply and four pieces of Band-Aid.

INSTRUCTION OUTFIT No. 25

This is an outfit of bandages, splints, tourniquet, etc., prepared for those who are called upon to give first aid instruction. The contents are intended to be used for illustrating and demonstrating first aid.

With the aid of this outfit, an instructor can precisely impart the essential features of first aid. It can be used with any system or text-book on first aid. It includes a syllabus of ten lessons based upon Johnson's Standard First Aid Manual.

BAND-AID

Band-Aid is a ready-to-use bandage for minor injuries—a combination of gauze pad and adhesive plaster. The gauze pad covers and

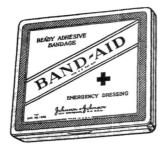

protects the wound, the adhesive plaster holds the pad in place.

The advantage of Band-Aid is that it makes possible a very quick application of a neat and clean bandage.

Band-Aid is a handy dressing to apply to the numerous cuts received by children at play and to the ordinary injuries incident to household or mechanical work. Numerous uses, such as protecting blisters on the feet, covering corns, protecting the hands of golfers, etc., will suggest themselves.

THE CONTENTS OF FIRST-AID OUTFITS

Following are brief descriptions of the principal items found in the various Johnson & Johnson first aid outfits:

FIRST AID FOR WOUNDS, PACKET No. 3

This packet is modeled after the famous First Help for Wounds packet used successfully in recent wars, and by all of the first aid and humane societies throughout the world. It is particularly adapted to factory injuries. The contents are as follows:

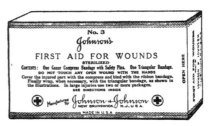

Gauze Bandage with compress attached, 4-inch pad, 72-inch tail. This bandage is for application to open wounds, for compression, for binding dressings and other purposes.

One Triangular Bandage, with illustrations showing use. Two safety pins. The whole is wrapped in an impermeable covering, enclosed in a cardboard carton, sterilized and sealed.

In military campaigns, in mining, forestry and camping, each person usually carries one of these packets in his pocket.

The value of the dressings in this packet has been well established, and it has been shown that they can be applied by any person without handling the wound, and that the dressing is just what is needed—an antiseptic, sterile dressing. In many instances the dressings found in this packet are sufficient for all purposes until the arrival of a surgeon.

It is difficult to imagine a wound or an injury which cannot be completely or properly dressed by the use of this First Aid for Wounds Packet. One or two packets are sufficient for the temporary dressing of an extensive injury.

ABSORBENT COTTON

This is a most useful article in the factory, shop, or household. Absorbent cotton does not mean ordinary cotton or cotton batting, but a specially prepared material whereby the elements in ordinary cotton (oil, wax and fat), which prevent absorption, are removed.

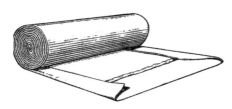

Absorbent cotton is by far the most generally used of all material for making compresses, for padding splints and slings, or for absorbing discharges, and is adaptable to every conceivable use.

In addition to its use as a wound dressing, as suggested throughout this Manual, absorbent cotton has a large use for mechanical, laboratory and household purposes.

Many kinds of so-called absorbent cotton are not suited for wound-dressing or other delicate purposes. Very often they are made in cotton mills of waste cotton; are filled with dirt, dust and leaves.

The Absorbent Cotton supplied in the outfits described in this Manual is known to surgeons as absolutely pure; that is to say, it is chemically pure and free from all foreign material. It is carefully cleansed and disinfected and subsequently sterilized within the package, and is, therefore, surgically clean. The cotton is rolled into layers or sheets with blue tissue paper between each of the layers and folded over the sides. It is wrapped in such

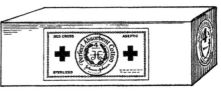

a way that all surfaces, including the edges, are fully protected from dust, dirt and infection, whether in or out of the carton. It can be cut or torn into any required shape.

SURGICAL GAUZE

This material, as its name indicates, is a thin, soft, woven cloth. For the purpose of covering a wound directly this gauze is, as a rule, a proper material to use. It absorbs very readily, contains no foreign matter, is soft and soothing and will form an easy, comfortable pressure and absorb all discharges and exudations. The packages of

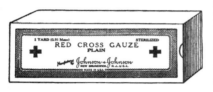

gauze supplied in the first aid outfits described in this Manual contain one square yard of surgical gauze, and this is used either whole or cut into suitable sizes or folded for making compresses, for covering large exposed sufaces, for applying dressings or solutions to burns or wounds. It may be adapted to innumerable conditions and circumstances.

Gauze cloth is a convenient material for use in the household, and should be substituted for all kinds of cloths, pads, bandages and compresses in the sick room, and used for dressing wounds and sores.

LINTON GAUZE BANDAGES

These bandages are absorbent, soft, and at the same time firm and strong. They are intended to be used as a direct covering for the wound. Their absorbency is useful to hold wound discharges. They are also useful in binding and holding other dressings and for the application of solutions and lotions to the wound. These gauze bandages are tightly rolled, and each bandage packed in a cardboard cylinder.

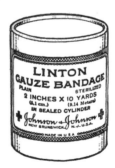

Special uses of the bandages are given in this Manual (see Bandaging).

COTTON ROLLER BANDAGES

These are ribbon-like strips of cotton cloth and are wound into cylinders.

They are strong and can therefore be used for binding up injuries in any part of the body.

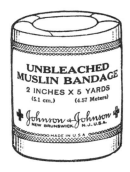

In general, these bandages are used to keep other dressings in place, to secure splints, to check bleeding, to protect the parts from external injury, to bind up fractures—in fact, their uses are innumerable and they may be said to be applicable to nearly every sort of injury.

Persons of ordinary intelligence can satisfactorily apply a roller bandage. Methods of application adapted to ordinary emergencies are described under the heading of "Bandaging" in this Manual.

COMPRESS BANDAGES

These gauze bandages, with a compress attached, have been called the most efficient first aid servants. A compress bandage is used to cover the wound and prevent hemorrhage. They are versatile and expedient.

ADHESIVE PLASTER

Rubber adhesive plaster, sometimes called surgeon's adhesive or adhesive tape, should be used instead of court or isinglass plaster as an application to wounds. It sticks without warming or other preparation. Its uses are too numerous to mention in this publication.

When the services of a physician can be secured, a layman should never attempt to apply adhesive plaster to a wounded surface. In applying adhesive plaster to a broken surface, the hands of the operator, the wound itself and the surrounding parts should be cleansed with an antiseptic soap, and made thoroughly dry with surgically clean gauze. The wound should never be entirely covered with adhesive plaster. The best method is to bring the surfaces together with narrow strips, leaving a space between each two strips for the wound to discharge.

When adhesive plaster is to be applied to a hairy part, the hair should be shaved off. No large open or raw surface should be covered with adhesive plaster. It should never be applied to burns.

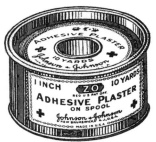

Adhesive plaster is very useful for holding dressings in place, when the patient is to be transported. Some of the more common applications for adhesive plaster are shown in the illustrations in this Manual.

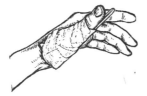
Fig. 118—Support for sprained thumb.

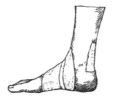
Fig. 119—Support for weak instep.

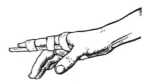
Fig. 120—Holding splint dressing for finger.

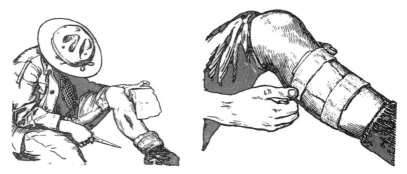
Figs. 121 and 122—Holding in place dressing of tear of leg.

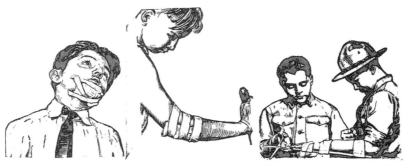
Fig. 123—Chin dressing.

Fig. 124—Elbow dressing.

Fig. 125—Holding simple splint dressing for arm.

The adhesive plaster sold under the name of "ZO" Adhesive Plaster is known to the surgical profession as a desirable form of adhesive plaster. It is applied without the aid of heat or moisture. It is non-irritating and will keep in any climate. It is supplied in various forms and sizes. A very convenient form of adhesive plaster for household use and for use in traveling, is the kind known as Zonas Adhesive Plaster. This plaster is in narrow widths one yard long, enclosed in a round metal case for the pocket.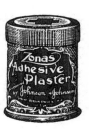

Non-Surgical Uses of Adhesive Plaster

Adhesive plaster has a great variety of uses independent of its surgical application, though the latter is the more important one.

It is a very useful article for mending clothing, furniture, and rubber articles such as water bags, syringes, hose, rain-coats, mackintoshes, boots, shoes and a thousand and one articles of the household. Anything made of rubber can be repaired, patched and rendered serviceable through its use.

Adhesive plaster is also used largely in making up and repairing electrical apparatus, as it is practically a non-conductor, is waterproof and adaptable to a variety of uses. Strips may be applied to the hands to prevent the action of caustic or corrosive liquids, and also to the finger in the form of a "finger cot."

It is most serviceable for the effectual closing of a room that is to be disinfected by vapors, such as sulphur fumes or formaldehyd gas. All cracks and crevices in the doors, windows, etc., are covered with narrow strips of plaster, and the room thus made vapor tight, whereas before the use of this substance, the escape of vapors in disinfecting was one of the weakest points of the process. This also suggests the use of the plaster as an emergency weather strip and to mend a broken window-pane.

The uses of adhesive plaster are almost without number. In all cases it makes a cheap, strong and durable binder so flexible that it will conform to the shape of any surface.

BURN DRESSING PACKET

This packet for burns holds four pieces of picric acid gauze, each about 18 inches square, and also an illustrated triangular bandage with two safety pins. It is absolutely complete in itself and offers a thoroughly reliable, efficient and speedy specific burn dressing. The contents are compressed and sealed in a strong carton, ready for use.

PETROLATUM

The chief use for which this article is placed in first aid outfits is as an application for burns.

The method of use is to cover the burned surface entirely with it, so as to exclude the air, and then to wrap the part thoroughly with surgical gauze. It is superior to oils and ordinary emollients by reason of its antiseptic properties.

It is supplied in two forms—carbolated, which contains carbolic acid, and in the form of an ointment made of petrolatum combined with bicarbonate of soda. The latter form is the preferred preparation for burns.

TOURNIQUET

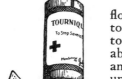

This simple device is designed to stop the profuse flow of blood from severed arteries in severe injuries to the limbs. It consists of a strong tape fastened to a wooden handle. The tape is to be wound once about the limb (between the heart and the injury) and passed through the slit in the handle, then under the handle. The handle is then twisted until sufficient pressure is applied to the artery to stop the blood spurt. The tourniquet should not be allowed to remain in place longer than is required to stop the blood flow, then loosened and retightened if necessary.

CAMPHENOL SOLUTION

This is an antiseptic for infected wounds. It is applied to wounds only after dilution with water.

Emergency dressings may be rendered antiseptic by dipping gauze or cotton in Camphenol solution and wringing out the excess fluid.

AROMATIC SPIRIT OF AMMONIA

There are occasions when the giving of a light stimulant is necessary, and for emergency use nothing is equal to aromatic spirit of ammonia. The dose is half a teaspoonful in half a glass or less of water and repeated in fifteen minutes if necessary, but not more than four doses. Stimulants, however, are only to be administered under the conditions stated in the Manual, or by direction of the physician.

SOLUTION OF IODINE

This is a solution of iodine of proper strength for application to wounds. In the first aid outfits it is supplied in vials, and also in tubes with swabs attached. A most convenient form is known as Ioply, each ampoule or small tube, with a swab attached, containing a supply sufficient to cover any ordinary wound.

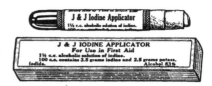

MERCUROCHROME SOLUTION

This is a solution of Mercurochrome, an antiseptic recommended as a substitute for iodine for application to open wounds. In the first aid outfits it is supplied in vials of appropriate size and also in ampoules, known as Mercuroply. Each Mercuroply contains an amount sufficient for every ordinary wound, and has a swab attached for application.

OTHER CONTENTS

Certain of the outfits also contain the following:

Wooden Splints: For supporting fractures. Particular uses are fully described in the Manual.

Boracic Acid Solution: For eye irritation and injuries.

Wooden Applicators: For the application of solutions to the eyes. Can also be used for painting parts with iodine, etc.

Tongue Depressors: For holding down the tongue in choking, drowning, etc.

Castor Oil: For application to the eye in the removal of foreign bodies, and for injuries to the eye.

Medicine Glass: For measuring and administering liquids

The cabinets and cases also contain safety pins, scissors and tweezers.

Each larger outfit contains a copy of the Standard First Aid Manual and each smaller cabinet contains full directions for the use of its contents.

FIRST AID SERVICE

Johnson & Johnson have instituted a First Aid Service Bureau, which fills a most important position in the world-wide First Aid movement.

The Service reaches beyond the production of outfits and supplies. It has assisted in the organization and installation of first aid systems in railways and transportation lines, factories and industries.

The bureau has been of special service to teachers and instructors in factories, mines, Y. M. C. A., Boy Scouts, Girl Scouts, and in other associations and organizations.

The Service is prepared to cooperate with all who may be interested in the subject of first aid.

In addition to the work of furnishing supplies and equipments there is issued by the Bureau a considerable amount of literature and other helps.

Persons interested in the promotion of first aid work or household hygiene in any capacity are invited to correspond with the Bureau.

Constructive literature covering the subject of first aid application, the care of the sick and the treatment of disease is cheerfully supplied. Write to Johnson & Johnson, New Brunswick, N. J.

FIRST AID CHART

Johnson's First Aid Chart covers the whole range of first aid, theory and practice, in picture and in text.

The chart is three-fold, lithographed in ten colors; the back is illustrated in black and white, and includes text matter giving complete instructions for the practical application of first aid.

It is at once a teaching chart and a practical guide for first aid work. It is an art creation, anatomically and scientifically correct. It is most complete, efficient and convenient, and opens a new chapter in the promulgation of first aid.

The subjects covered by the chart are as follows:

Bleeding
Course of the main arteries of the body
Practical methods of arresting bleeding
Fractures
Sprains, strains and other injuries
Practical emergency methods of applying splints
Uses of the Triangular and Roller bandages
Fainting
Wound dressing

Shock
Burns and scalds
Railroad and machinery accidents
Foreign bodies in the eye, ear, nose and throat
Sunstroke
Heat prostration
Suffocation
Electricity accidents
Insensibility
Drowning
Artificial respiration
Poisons and antidotes

This chart will at once appeal to the doctor, the nurse, the instructor in first aid and to the lay student.

For schools, gymnasiums, railways, mines, first aid teams and crews, industrial plants, manufacturing institutions and everywhere that first aid is practiced, taught or studied, this chart will be of great utility. It is a complete guide to first aid that anybody can use who can understand a picture.

For illustration of this chart see the opposite page.

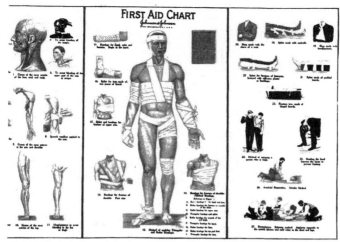

First Aid Chart, size 27 x 44 inches, mounted on heavy board. Folds for carrying. The front is in ten colors. The back contains full first aid instructions in black and white.

INDEX